PRAISE FOR

TEACHING YOGA BEYOND THE POSES, VOLUME 2

"*Teaching Yoga Beyond the Poses, Volume 2* is a book that seamlessly blends the ancient wisdom of yoga with modern insights. It's not just a guide, it's an inspiration that encourages a deeper understanding of core yoga principles. From insightful reflections on Patanjali to Hindu mythology, asana, and other timeless yoga themes, this book offers numerous points of study and reflection. Its holistic approach reminds you that yoga is more than asana. This book is a beacon of light for teachers of all traditions, inspiring them to delve deeper into the rich philosophy of yoga."

—GABRIELLE HARRIS, author of *The Language of Yin* and *The Inspired Yoga Teacher*

"Two essential parts of translating the teachings of the ancient path of yoga are clarity and accessibility. Yoga students and teachers often desire to understand how to apply the teachings to their lives, communities, and the greater world. Sage and Alexandra have written a comprehensive, relatable guide meeting this desire. Through their own stories, deep study of the path, and sharing of resources and templates for themes, they have created a guide that will support teachers in facilitating the practice of yoga in an authentic, meaningful, and inspiring way. *Teaching Yoga Beyond the Poses, Volume 2* illustrates how the path of yoga is meant to change us as teachers, guides, and facilitators; in turn, we can change and transform others through offering teachings from the path."

—MICHELLE JOHNSON, author of *Skill in Action* and *Illuminating Our True Nature*

"This treasure trove of a book will be an invaluable resource for yoga teachers looking for inspiration to uplift their teaching. Sage Rountree and Alexandra DeSiato generously share their wisdom and experience in a way that empowers the reader to connect with their own inner wisdom and gain confidence in their ability to teach engaging and inspiring yoga sessions. This book is a must-read for both new and experienced yoga teachers alike."

—JILLY SHIPWAY, author of *Yoga Through the Year*

"I love this book. It's a game changer for any of us looking for new, innovative, and inspiring ways to weave the deeper teachings of yoga into an often fast-paced, body-based practice. Sage Rountree and Alexandra DeSiato have wisely and lovingly presented 54 new themes—ranging from ancient to contemporary, from spiritual to the ordinary—that will allow us to teach with clarity, confidence, and authenticity, and in doing so, hopefully awaken within our students the desire to apply these teachings to their own lives."

—LINDA SPARROWE, former editor-in-chief of *Yoga International* and author of *Yoga at Home* and coauthor of *The Woman's Book of Yoga and Health*

"May I be the first to proclaim that *Teaching Yoga Beyond the Poses* has started a movement? Every time I teach a workshop, yoga teachers tell me how much this book has become their bible. This second volume is full of confidence-building inspiration. If you want to find a way to address real-life concerns through a yogic lens, this book is for you. If you want to find a way to share your personal yoga epiphanies in a way that touches your students, this book is for you. Yoga is vast. *Teaching Yoga Beyond the Poses, Volume 2* offers yoga teachers direction and inspiration for how to shape, organize, and clearly share their wisdom in their yoga classes."

—CYNDI LEE, author of *May I Be Happy* and *Drip Drip Drip, the Bucket Fills* on substack

"*Teaching Yoga Beyond the Poses, Volume 2* is a must-have resource for all yoga teachers. This book not only gives you step-by-step instructions for how to find your voice, easily theme your classes, and take your teaching to the next level, but you'll learn how to truly add impact and meaning for your students and go deeper into your own practice as well. This book is a game changer in the yoga world and needs to be mandatory reading for all yoga teachers."

—MARY OCHSNER, founder of the Yoga+ by Mary app

TEACHING

YOGA

BEYOND

THE

POSES

VOLUME 2

Also by Sage Rountree and Alexandra DeSiato

Teaching Yoga Beyond the Poses

Lifelong Yoga

TEACHING YOGA BEYOND THE POSES

VOLUME 2

54 NEW THEMES, TEMPLATES, AND IDEAS FOR INTEGRATING INSPIRATION INTO YOUR CLASS

SAGE ROUNTREE AND **ALEXANDRA DESIATO**

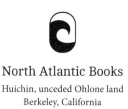

North Atlantic Books
Huichin, unceded Ohlone land
Berkeley, California

Published by
North Atlantic Books
Huichin, unceded Ohlone land
Berkeley, California

Cover photo © Natalia via Getty Images
Cover design by Jasmine Hromjak and Rob Johnson
Book design by Happenstance Type-O-Rama
Illustrations by Lasha Mutual, https://lashamutual.com

Printed in the United States of America

Teaching Yoga Beyond the Poses, Volume 2: 54 New Themes, Templates, and Ideas for Integrating Inspiration into Your Class is sponsored and published by North Atlantic Books, an educational nonprofit based in the unceded Ohlone land Huichin (Berkeley, CA) that collaborates with partners to develop cross-cultural perspectives; nurture holistic views of art, science, the humanities, and healing; and seed personal and global transformation by publishing work on the relationship of body, spirit, and nature.

MEDICAL DISCLAIMER: The following information is intended for general information purposes only. Individuals should always see their health care provider before administering any suggestions made in this book. Any application of the material set forth in the following pages is at the reader's discretion and is their sole responsibility.

North Atlantic Books's publications are distributed to the US trade and internationally by Penguin Random House Publisher Services. For further information, visit our website at www.northatlanticbooks.com.

Library of Congress Cataloging-in-Publication Data

Names: Rountree, Sage Hamilton, author. | Desiato, Alexandra, 1979– author.
Title: Teaching yoga beyond the poses : a practical workbook for integrating themes, ideas, and inspiration into your class / Sage Rountree and Alexandra DeSiato.
Description: Berkeley, California : North Atlantic Books, [2019]
Identifiers: LCCN 2018048512 | ISBN 9781623173227 (paperback)
Subjects: LCSH: Hatha yoga—Study and teaching. | BISAC: HEALTH & FITNESS / Yoga. | BODY, MIND & SPIRIT / Meditation. | SELF-HELP / Motivational & Inspirational.
Classification: LCC RA781.7 .R72 2019 | DDC 613.7/046076—dc23
LC record available at https://lccn.loc.gov/2018048512

ISBN 979-8-88984-195-1 (pbk.) — ISBN 979-8-88984-196-8 (ebook)

1 2 3 4 5 6 7 8 9 KPC 30 29 28 27 26 25

To our readers

CONTENTS

PREFACE

The popularity of *Teaching Yoga Beyond the Poses* was no surprise to us, although it was a delight. We have long seen that students and yoga teachers are eager to imbue their practice with meaning and to have a framework to do so. Since the book became available in May 2019, we've only seen this desire grow in the yoga community. Readers of *Teaching Yoga Beyond the Poses* are passionate about how meaningful the book has been for them. We see this in Amazon and Goodreads comments and ratings; on social media, where we love seeing your photos of the book, dogeared and covered in notes; and in successful theming workshops based on the book that we have led at Carolina Yoga Company in North Carolina and the Kripalu Center for Yoga and Health in Massachusetts. Readers and teachers love the book, but they are still seeking guidance. That is why this book has been such a success—and why it is time for the next iteration of this concept.

This new companion volume, with all new material, continues to build on the initial purpose of the book: to offer teachers and students evergreen guided and ready-made inspirational messages that they can both use as-is and also mold into their own, so they can serve their own students best. Like its predecessor, we hope this book will help teachers refine their voice, teach with confidence, and feel both inspired and inspirational. And we hope it will give students insight into how classes are planned, how yoga comes to life on and off the mat, and how their practice can help them live a fulfilled life.

Another reason we are revisiting the topic of theming yoga classes: we know yoga philosophy is applicable to our daily lives. Just like the physical practice of yoga, yoga's philosophical concepts and spiritual inquires can help us find deeper connection to ourselves. Not only do we want *you* to find a richer relationship with yoga by better understanding and applying some of the essential themes and philosophies to yourself, we also want you to feel empowered to bring these ideas to your students. The result for you and your students is transformative.

Just as the poses themselves are not something sacred or owned by a select few teachers, yoga's suggestions for how to live a more blissful life and move toward greater liberation are not ideas to be gatekept from your students, but shared. You do not have to be a yoga scholar to share what you've learned, and if this book helps you find the words to do so and the confidence to know that the message you share matters, we have done what we set out to do. The point is that you offer your students guidance as they navigate not just yoga's poses but so much more beyond the poses too.

ACKNOWLEDGMENTS

Thanks to you, the reader, for your presence and attention. Your enthusiasm about the first volume of this book has delighted us and spurred this new volume. We are so grateful.

Thanks to our agent, Linda Konner. Thanks to the team at North Atlantic Books: to Susan Bumps for planting this idea in our heads; to Shayna Keyles for her early support of the project and for welcoming a new second volume; to Margeaux Weston for shepherding the book through its first draft; to production editor Janelle Ludowise for running from there; to copy editor Christopher Church for keeping it clean; to proofreader Rebecca Rider for buffing it to a shine; to art director Jasmine Hromjak and typesetter Kate Kaminski for dressing it up beautifully.

Special thanks to Lasha Mutual for contributing her art to this volume. Lasha, your practice shines through in your work! We are so glad to have your illustrations illuminate these messages.

Thanks to our students both at Carolina Yoga and around the country, for being careful listeners and for sharing with us what they take away from the messages we offer. Y'all have contributed immensely to the power of these books.

Thanks most of all to our families and to our special partnership that makes completing projects like this feel like less than half the work—and more than double the fun.

PART I

OUR THEMING APPROACH

1

WHERE WE BEGAN

Writing *Teaching Yoga Beyond the Poses* felt like writing a theming manual for ourselves. As teachers who had been through numerous yoga teacher trainings, who had taught numerous trainings, and who had years of experience teaching yoga classes, writing books on specific aspects of yoga, and sharing workshops on how yoga can serve particular populations, we arrived at a place where we wanted to better articulate how yoga had started to elevate us as human beings. And we knew if we—as seasoned teachers—were still trying to untangle how to do that authentically, humbly, and also with authority, we guessed that other teachers might feel the same way. Our template helped us see how we could take ideas that felt transformative and illuminating to us and share them with our students in a way they could grasp and digest, all in the context of a physical movement class.

We think this is why it resonated with teachers: on some level, regardless of how many years they had under their belts, previous trainings had not yet equipped them to speak confidently to their students about ancient or esoteric ideas.

THOUGHTFUL THEMING GROWS YOUR SELF-CONFIDENCE

The energy you bring to your classroom is transmitted to your students. It affects them. The more relaxed you feel as you lead a class, the more relaxing it is in turn for the students. Building your confidence in every element of classroom management, then, is the key to relaxing—and to teaching a class that leaves your students happily centered and calm, no matter the format.

Nowhere are we less confident than when talking about philosophy. Often this is because it either seems too esoteric and lofty, or because, at the other end of the spectrum, it feels too personal. We want to help you find the middle path, where your message is both universal and specific, and where you feel confident about delivering it clearly.

Knowing that you can lead others through choreographed movements while helping them notice and utilize their breathing and while *also* offering them a perspective shift on their lives—that's powerful stuff. Speaking with authority about conceptual, spiritual ideas will make you a better teacher in general, even though, frankly, initially talking about this stuff can feel strange and stilted. Once you manage to find your voice to present philosophical materials in a way that resonates with others, the rest comes a bit easier. You stand at the front of your class with more confidence. You lead the entire practice with greater authority to be in the role of the teacher.

A DESIRE FOR GREATER MEANING

There's a lovely Philip Larkin poem called "Church Going" where the narrator ruminates on the staying power of religious faith. Toward the end of the poem, he decides that churches will likely remain in use indefinitely, "since someone will forever be surprising / A hunger in himself to be more serious." You may have noticed this same desire in yourself—a hunger to be more serious and to learn more from yoga than just the poses, transitions, and common sequences. And you correctly recognized this same desire for greater meaning in your students. A point that we'll never tire of making is that your students are coming to yoga, not barre or Pilates or HIIT. They are coming to move, breathe, *and* to make space for a deeper connection to their spiritual selves. Advanced practitioners may recognize that and give voice to it by picking up this book, or *Teaching Yoga Beyond the Poses,* or any number of books that offer translations of the ancient texts of yoga. Newer students come to yoga with this hunger and desire too, even if they can't quite name it or explain it.

Have you noticed that students often gravitate to yoga when their lives are in flux? Or, if you went through a yoga teacher training program, there are probably reasons related to transition, deepening your own practice, and life changes that brought you there. We also see this in Alexandra's prenatal yoga classes, where many students are coming to yoga for the first time, searching for something grounding amid an incredibly unmooring life shift. Many students are coming to yoga hungry for more meaning, more self-knowledge, and perspective-shifting lessons that help them navigate the uncharted waters of their very existence.

Or, as a student of yoga, maybe you were drawn to it first as a physical movement practice. Floating through vinyasas felt good! The joy of lifting into an arm balance felt powerful. The release of Savasana was full-body sweetness. But over time, you started noticing that the chanting, intention-setting, and ritual parts of yoga spoke to you too. You got more and more curious about the origins of yoga, about its ancient texts, about the lineage of some of the practices. You wanted to know more about what the other aspects of yoga could offer you on your life path. That's certainly been our journey. And it's your students' journeys too.

We live in a world that moves extremely quickly. There is constant change and immediate access to information, all of which can be dysregulating. If the experience of a well-themed class can offer students a bit of a life raft in the unmooring waters of our modern world, then you are doing more than affecting individuals; you're contributing to a collective calm and groundedness, a universal slowing-down that humanity as a whole is desperate for.

·············· YOUR VOICES BRING US JOY! ··············

There is hardly anything better than serving in a role of mentorship and seeing what others are capable of doing even before they see it. This is incredibly gratifying in one-on-one mentorship roles, but because of social media and interconnectedness, so many of you have reached out to us to share the themes from *Teaching Yoga Beyond the Poses* you're using and the themes you've felt inspired to bring to your students—and to share your students' responses to your gentle words, enthusiastic inspiration, and greater presence. Every Instagram post and story we're tagged in, every email we receive, every Facebook yoga teachers group that shouts out our book as a helpful tool for stepping into the role of the teacher has felt like a moment of mentorship. Know that when we see that, we celebrate with each other that your voices are showing up louder and more confidently in the world. For us, it has been gratifying beyond words to see you shine as teachers and share your wisdom and perspective with others, even when it made you a little nervous at first to do so.

Perhaps because so many yoga teachers are women, this has also felt like some sweet feminist empowerment too. We obviously love seeing all teachers grow, but it feels personally relatable to see women yoga teachers (yoginis!) grow in their sense of self-confidence, self-kindness, and leadership. So often women cap off their brilliant ideas with a disclaimer that lightly denigrates. Even adding something like, "Does that make sense?" suggests on some level that the speaker is insecure about her voice. But as you have learned already, or will continue to learn as you carry on your theming journey, there is no room for "Does that make sense?" in the role of the teacher. When you stand confidently and share an idea that you relate to, understand, and want your students to feel or grapple with, you know it makes sense. You stand at the front of the room with greater ease and certainty, and that self-assurance carries into all aspects of your life. We love to see it.

·········· WHAT WE HEAR READERS SAY ··········

What a treat it has been to watch *Teaching Yoga Beyond the Poses* grow a life and community of its own! We are so grateful to every reader who has reviewed the book, posted about it, shared it with friends, and told us how it has helped you. We sure hope you'll be equally vociferous in talking about volume 2.

One takeaway we hear from your feedback is that you are cherry-picking, pulling out what worked from our suggestions, leaving what doesn't resonate with you, and making these theme ideas and templates your own. This is just what we'd hoped for. We understand that you may not use our suggested quotes, chants, and songs, but that you feel empowered to choose your own.

We both vividly recall an online review of the first book that fixated on one suggested song. The reviewer made it abundantly clear they would never play that song in a yoga class. Great! That's the point. When you read our suggestions and have a visceral response either way—loving an idea or disliking it—you've done important work in uncovering your authentic voice for sharing ideas. We know it is equally valuable for you to deeply embrace one of our suggestions and also to thoroughly reject another. In either moment, your authority as a teacher who trusts their voice is growing, and our work is having exactly the impact we'd hoped. This makes us feel like yoga aunties in the best way—we shared some wisdom that we have learned, both through our teachers and our lived experience, and in turn it has helped you.

Better yet, we hear that your students appreciate the lessons you are bringing to them. This makes us feel like great aunts, like useful crones. And we love knowing that when you are inspiring your students, your classes grow. As your classes grow, your confidence as a teacher builds, creating a self-sustaining momentum that benefits your career and your students' practices in deep ways. What a win-win.

Best of all, our takeaway from your embrace of the first volume and the workshops we've led: You recognize your role as a teacher goes beyond just offering sequences and poses. You are, in effect, a spiritual guide. That doesn't need to be a scary thing. You are lay clergy in a philosophical and secularly spiritual practice. You are sharing the wisdom of your own experience in ways that helps your students alleviate their own suffering. When you do this, you see your role in yoga as so much more than guiding the physical practice. As a consequence, your own relationship to yoga—and to your role as a human living here and now—deepens. What a wonderful journey!

2

WHERE WE ARE HEADING

We have several goals for this new book: first, we want to offer you more of what was useful about *Teaching Yoga Beyond the Poses*—more themes, more self-reflection, more exposure to yogic philosophy, and more helpful ideas about what it means to be human. We're also excited to share how our approach to theming has evolved in the five years since we wrote *Teaching Yoga Beyond the Poses*. We're eager to share new ideas we have on how you can further weave your messages into your students' lives off the mat. Finally, we want to give you more opportunity to explore your voice, so you'll find more journaling prompts here in part 3. It may be helpful to keep this self-reflection close to your vest, but note that we are always happy to chat with you on social media or through our online course at https://teachingyogabeyondtheposes.com. You're not alone on this journey of self-reflection and *svadhyaya*.

And, of course, in this next iteration of our ideas on theming (which, with great amusement, we referred to as *2 Beyond 2 Poses* and other variations on the *Fast & Furious* movie franchise titles until we settled on the current title), we are excited to share more theme ideas we've personally been teaching, talking about, and ruminating on.

MORE THEMES, MORE FURIOUS

We love creating themes, and we're excited to bring you fifty-four more fleshed-out themes in this new volume. Some of these new themes are based in classical yoga tradition, including the ancient texts of yoga, the Tantric embodiment of masculine and feminine, and Indian mythology, imagery, and stories. Here's some history that you likely already know: Yoga is quite old. Scholars and historians don't know exactly how old, since for much of yoga's existence it was passed on from teacher to students in an oral tradition. And what was passed on wasn't the poses, which for the most part came much later in yoga's history. Instead, what was passed on were ideas on living well and instructions, sometimes about meditation, ritual, and breathwork, for how to suffer less and how to move toward greater spiritual liberation.

One book of such instructions is the Yoga Sutras. In the sutras, the sage Patanjali offers short aphorisms for how someone on the path of yoga might choose to behave, what they might prioritize, and what the expected outcomes will be if they stay on the path. Some of it is very accessible for modern-day readers, and there are plenty of excellent translations of this text that extrapolate on each sutra. Some of the sutras get . . . uh, weird—which brings us to a helpful point about all yoga, whether it's the physical poses or the historical teachings. It's not a religion, and it's not a dogmatic spiritual practice. (What's the adage? Anyone saying otherwise is trying to sell you something—probably their brand of yoga, or some really flashy leggings.) Ultimately you get to take from yoga what you find useful, and that's true of historical tomes like the Yoga Sutras. And you get to leave the parts that don't resonate in our modern world, that seem needlessly complicated, or that you don't connect to. In his seminal text *The Heart of Yoga,* T. K. V. Desikachar (the son of Tirumalai Krishnamacharya, who is widely considered one of the most important figures in the modern resurgence of yoga and is in part responsible for its growth to the West) says, "Yoga is not fixed. Yoga is a creation. I know the way you teach will be different from the way that I teach, and the way I teach is different from the way my father taught." In this way, he acknowledges that yoga is ever-evolving, and that it's shaped appropriately by each teacher who offers it to others. Specifically about the Yoga Sutras, he says an important message from it is that "Each person gets different things from the same teaching based on his or her own perspective. There is nothing wrong with this. This is how it is."*

---

* T. K. V. Desikachar, *The Heart of Yoga: Developing a Personal Practice* (Rochester, VT: Inner Traditions International, 1995), xxvi.

In our themes in this book, we're sharing some selections from the sutras that we love, that have spoken to us, and that offer something resonant for modern existence. Some of them may be familiar to you from your studies, but some may not be. In either case, we hope our suggestions of how to offer these pieces of yoga wisdom as themes in movement classes land with you and are helpful. And we hope our theming on these few sutras inspires you to continue your studies of this valuable yogic text and to revisit it to find more gems of ancient wisdom to relay to your students in the present day.

You'll also find theming on the archetypes of the divine masculine and feminine, embodied in Shiva and Shakti. The duality of masculine Shiva and feminine Shakti coming together to form a whole, a union, a nondual divine likely originates in Tantric yoga philosophy, but it may predate that. Because yoga has been around for so long, it weaves through hundreds of years of Indian philosophy, Hinduism, and Buddhism—and often, ideas from all of these philosophical and religious paths overlap and intersect with one another. In Tantric yogic cosmology, which informs our modern Hatha practice of yoga, both masculine and feminine are equally divine. The goddess depicted in various forms or the divine feminine is of particular importance in Tantric yoga philosophy, making it relevant to the matriarchal slant we see in modern-day yoga leadership.

Shiva, the divine masculine, and Shakti, the divine feminine, are in a constant play together. In Tantric philosophy, this play is called Lila, and it is the basis of all of creation and existence. These masculine and feminine are archetypes, not to be taken literally. There are stereotypical and mythical attributes assigned to these archetypes that might seem dated in the twenty-first-century West, with our recognition that gender identity may be in constant flux and genders may be claimed and expressed far outside the binary. In some ways, though, we can conceive of Shiva and Shakti not as separate entities of gender but as poles at either end of a very broad, fascinating, and curious spectrum, where just about every permutation of gendered experience can live. And as poles on the gender spectrum, they point to some universal experiences. If we only perceive them as "male" and "female" rather than expressions of gender that may show up in anyone's lived experience, they might seem out of sync with the times. Instead, we can imagine Shiva or Shakti as energetic experiences that any and all beings can have, whatever gender they know themselves to be.

As we've already noted, and as your own studies of the history of yoga have no doubt revealed to you, yoga philosophy grew up not just alongside but threaded through and affected by Hindu mythology and stories. That's why we see so many poses inspired by the powerful deities that pervade that faith. For our themes, we've looked at some of our favorite mystical stories through the lens of yoga. And while we've gleaned the wisdom of only a few parables and stories here, stories from the Hindu canon offer rich and compelling explorations in a yoga class. If this is a line of thinking you'd love to pursue as you continue to build your own themes, you'll find book recommendations at the start of each chapter, where we highlight other sources of inspiration.

It's worth noting, and it's something we pointed to in our first book, that we think *all* faith traditions offer relevant themes for modern living, and in the spirit of spiritual study and exploration, you should expose yourself to the divine and mystical wherever it presents itself. You might consider sacred texts of any faith that speak to you as part of your tool kit for theming. There is a tremendous difference between sharing an element of a faith as a theme and serving as a representative of, promoting, or proselytizing for the religion it comes from. For example, you may offer themes on the practice of atonement present in various religious faiths and sects without formally celebrating a specific holiday or advocating a religious practice.

While many of the themes on offer in this volume are derived from ancient sources, some emerge more from the ways yoga is practiced in the twenty-first-century West. We have a series of themes we call "simple but profound," which are lessons that are exactly that—they'll resonate with your students, no intellectual discourse or mental gymnastics required. Many of our themes may be familiar to you. Here, our goal is to elevate simple or familiar themes so they are freshly resonant for you and your students.

In keeping with the spirit of yoga as a pathway for everyone—an evolution that occurred in the history of the practice as it went from being something for only the most ascetic upper-class men to what it is today, a practice for everyone—we also have themes that invoke yoga as a vehicle for social justice. Certainly talking about social justice isn't the same as taking action. But within the context of a single yoga class, sharing thoughts on social justice is what you *can* do, and we encourage you to do so.

One useful strategy to bring activism to your yoga teaching off the mat includes offering reparations discounts to Black, brown, and Indigenous people and other people of color, and to offer gratitude discounts to students of Indian or South Asian descent. We offer this at Sage's studio in the yoga teacher training that Alexandra leads, and it can be a vital way to put your money where your mouth is when it comes to social justice work. In our themes on social justice, our approach is helping you speak to these topics in a way that considers you may not be a representative of the groups you are advocating for—both a powerful and also a tenuous place to be.

Finally, one of the groups of themes we are most excited to share are lessons from our students, including you! We have heard so many beautiful themes and lessons from the students in our general classes; from the teachers who join us on retreat and workshop weekends in our home studio in Carrboro, North Carolina, at Kripalu Center for Yoga and Health, and elsewhere; and through your generous sharing on social media of the themes you created.

····· OUR THEMING APPROACH, EVOLVED ·····

If you've read volume 1 of *Teaching Yoga Beyond the Poses,* and especially if you've used its template to write your own themes, you'll notice that we have made some upgrades to the original template. Here's what we are doing differently in volume 2, and why. As with everything we offer, we invite you to try on this new, expanded template, and then to make choices that work best for your teaching style and your students' needs.

The evolutions in our template here reflect the evolution in our approach to theming and our own teaching growth. Since we wrote *Teaching Yoga Beyond the Poses* and began paying close attention to how themes land in class, as well as listening to other teachers' experiences, we added some cues to be sure you are centering the student experience and not your own. We know your classes will benefit from this, as will you, because it means you don't need to be the center of attention. Instead, how your students relate to the theme is what matters. And each student can have their own unique relationship to the message—that's their job to create, not yours.

The headings here reflect the prompts in our template, and beneath each we explain how you can use the prompts to develop a roadmap for your class theme. You can find downloadable templates in various file formats at https://teaching yogabeyondtheposes.com.

Expound on Your Theme and Connect It to a Personal and a Universal Experience

The major lesson we've been offering as we teach others to theme classes is to find a way to make each theme both personal and universal—both specific and broad. Finding this balance is key. Illustrating how the theme applies to you personally as the teacher gives the theme weight and gives you authority as a speaker. This is a rhetorical device called *ethos*, which means the argument depends on the credibility of the speaker. It can humanize something that seems to belong to the lofty realms of philosophy or the dusty domains of obscure sacred texts. By adding your personal story to an esoteric idea, you can guide your students to the theme through the lens of your own experience. But be careful to do this only when it is applicable and comfortable. Trying to crowbar a personal story into a message can ring false, and it risks making you seem like an egotist who needs the attention of the class as a power play. You'll find more on storytelling in the next chapter.

In addition to encouraging you to make the universal personal and the personal universal while introducing your theme at the start of class, we have added a suggestion that you offer reflection time for your students to look backward and forward, considering how the theme relates to their own lives. This helps decenter your own story and subjecthood. It takes the focus off you as the teacher, so that each student is able to focus on how the message applies to their own unique lived experience. Give students space and time for meditative self-study in your class. We know that is where much of the deep learning of yoga happens: not in a pose, necessarily, but in witnessing the internal monologue that happens as ideas are processed either in stillness or in motion. Practically, that means you offer cues to your students to turn in and meditate on the theme you've offered. You ask rhetorical questions so they can see the theme in application to their lived experience.

This approach harks back to a useful reflective model that asks, "What? So what? Now what?" The "What?" is your presentation of the theme and its central message, with both specific and general—or personal and universal—examples. The "So what?" is your invitation, issued early in the class, that students consider how this idea resonates with their own lives. And the "Now what?" is your prompt, given late in the class, that students think about how this will play out in their lives in the future and outside the yoga studio. In our template, the "What?" goes under the expounding on the theme, the "So what?" is included in things to say at the start of class, and the "Now what?" comes at the close of class, either en route to final relaxation or on the way out.

Chants, Quotes, Mantras, Poems, or Songs That Connect

These clearly reflect our tastes. We've noted what is a poem and what is a song, so there's no detective work needed. You'll likely have lots to add. Please do! We'd love for you to share your suggestions with us using the hashtag #teachingyogabeyond theposes, or send us a message at https://teachingyogabeyondtheposes.com. At the website, you'll also find a playlist with all our suggested songs and links to the poems we reference.

It is never the case that you have to offer a poem, mantra, or quote to your students or play music in class. These are just more options for ways you can bring your theme to life and move ideas from abstract to concrete.

Practices That Work with Your Theme

Volume 1 suggested poses or transitions that might work with each theme. Here, we're using a broader term, *practices,* to encompass not only poses and transitions but perhaps also *pranayama, kriyas, mudras,* and anything else that makes sense to you. We hope that your teaching continues to evolve too, and that you include elements of yoga beyond asana.

Distill Your Theme to a Short Sentence or Intention

This prompt encourages you to rephrase the theme in your own words. It might take the form of a sentence or even just a phrase. You could invite students to adopt this phrase as their intention for the class, if they don't have an intention already set. This could be a phrase that you use throughout the practice, remembering that repetition is an important part of theming.

Phrases or Sentences to Employ in These Parts of Your Class

As in volume 1, we make suggestions for what you might say about your theme before, during, and after your class, both in movement and in stillness. This is the sign of a master themer: they don't just mention the theme once, but instead work it through every element of the entire practice, start, middle, and end. It's critical that you fulfill any expectations you establish at the start. This yields a satisfying experience for your students. The Russian playwright Anton Chekhov famously taught that any element introduced at the beginning of a play—he used a loaded gun as his example—must be there for a reason; if there is no reason, it should be cut. If you've followed a long-running television show, go back and watch the first episode. In prestige dramas, you'll find many of the themes of the entire series are laid out in the pilot. And in network shows, often you find that characters—even the actors playing them—are often jettisoned sometime after the pilot, which is often shot on spec long before the show is ordered as a full series. You can avoid this unsatisfying approach by thinking through what you'll say at the start and end of class, and what you'll say during movement and in stillness.

Many of our suggestions of things to say during class are phrased as questions. Open-ended questions allow your students to answer in their own minds. As students consider and come to realize what they think, they are engaging in the silent half of a dialogue with you. Questions also have a way of catching attention more than statements do, and for this reason, questions serve to bring your students into the present. If they have wandered off in their minds back to a work email or some other distraction, a question like, "Can you breathe more fully here?" brings them back to the present moment. They think, "Well, *can* I breathe more fully here?" And then they do.

And this is a critical point: Teaching a class is having a conversation with your students. But their side of the conversation happens nonverbally. They are responding to your statements, questions, and prompts with their bodies and minds. But you don't get to hear these replies out loud. This can take some getting used to. Often your own anxious mind puts words in your students' mouths, assigning value to their expressions. This is a dangerous trip down a very slippery slope. Someone's thinking face, or their careful listening face, might read to you like repulsion, boredom, or frustration. As best you can, try not to let it. Trust in your message, and in your students' ability to process it in their own time, regardless of what their facial expressions seem to be telling you. Consider the central message of one of the most important texts in yoga, the Bhagavad Gita: Do your duty with no attachment to result. Your actions are within your control. Your students' responses to your class and theming are not.

Keep in mind that all of this theming talk is equal in importance to contemplative silence. Don't keep up a running commentary at the expense of giving your students plenty of quiet time and space to process your message and how it relates to their experience. Speak to offer instruction and share a message; don't speak to fill space.

OPENING

Here's where you'll ask students to reflect on the theme and how it applies to their own lived experience ("So what?"). You could also invite them to explore the theme during class. This looking backward can come right after your introduction of the theme. Say something like, "Take a moment to remember a time in your life when something similar happened. What did you learn? How does this concept illuminate that experience for you? And how might you like to explore this idea as we move and breathe together today?"

DURING MOVEMENTS

This is your chance to apply the theme to the physical aspects of class. Sometimes, messages land best during a pivotal moment: in a harder transition, before or after a tricky balance pose, after your class has tried a new approach to a familiar asana. Consider when your words may have the greatest effect.

DURING PAUSES

What you say during pauses can lead students to consider how your idea interacts with their attitudes and mindsets. We find these considerations can be especially powerful. Be sure to leave time for students to silently process as they rest—don't narrate the entire experience.

CLOSING

The close of class is your opportunity to restate your theme, like the finale of a symphony ties up all the motifs it has laid out.

Just as we want you to have students reflect on your theme in the context of their past experiences, we now suggest that near the end of class you give students a moment to look ahead. This is the "Now what?" Invite them to think about how this theme will manifest in their lives in the near future. This is the pivotal moment where your students see the theme move from the microcosm of their practice life to the macrocosm of their life off the mat. What you say here can help your students better live their yoga.

These closing remarks on your theme can happen at various times: during the wind-down prior to Savasana, before moving out of Savasana, while students rest on their sides en route to sitting up, in sitting at the close of class. In this way, you're offering students a chance to build life skills and to walk off the mat better prepared to meet the moment.

Takeaway Ideas

We use the term *takeaway* to refer to a physical or virtual lagniappe that you offer your students—something that points back to your theme. *Lagniappe* is a word that means "a little extra gift"; it comes from the Quechua language via Spanish. It's often used in the context of restaurant hospitality. If you're of a certain age of Food Network fandom, you might remember hearing Emeril Lagasse say the word frequently on his cooking shows ("Bam!"). In the restaurant world, a lagniappe is a gift from the kitchen. It could be an amuse-bouche, a little gift to stimulate your taste buds and make you smile, but it could also be something later in the meal, like a bonus side or a cordial sent over with your dessert. A lagniappe can also be a little gift with a purchase at a retail store, something to sweeten the memory of an exchange.

Consider adding a takeaway lagniappe for your students. This could be as simple as a card or a slip of paper with your quote or the chant used in class. Or it could be more elaborate: a recording of a meditation, or a robust email newsletter with an essay, quotes, and playlist. The sky—and your studio policies around contact with students; see the explanation in "Nonsolicitation Policies" below—is the limit here. Your lagniappe can fit whatever your creativity comes up with, and whatever feels most authentic to you.

Students *love* getting a lagniappe. First, it shows the care you have put into planning the class. You weren't winging it or making it up as you went along. Instead, you clearly took the time to think through your message and carefully design your class. Even a simple slip of paper with a printed or handwritten quote set up at each mat space, or placed there during Savasana, is evidence of how seriously you take your job as leader of your class. It is a sign of hospitality that goes a long way toward making students feel welcome, comfortable, and cared for.

A lagniappe is a way for students to take yoga off the mat and into their daily lives. Students report placing quote or chant cards in their wallets, on a mirror at home, or on their dashboard to remind themselves of the lesson they learned. Perfect! This is taking yoga beyond the poses and into the world. The more your students can learn to apply yoga's lessons off the mat, the more they can have a positive effect in the students' lives—and the lives of everyone they touch throughout the day. While some of the takeaways we offer in the themes here might be elaborate in a regular weekly class, they are a wonderful way to add value and intentionality to your workshops, which can also be themed just like your classes.

Your lagniappe could, then, be a physical copy of the quote or chant you used in class. Or it could be a prompt for journaling keyed to the reflection you introduced during class. This is a way to encourage your students to meditate and reflect on yoga's lessons outside the class context. Doing so is the best first step toward deepening the practice.

Another great lagniappe is sharing recordings to follow along with. This doesn't need to be a video of your full class—not only is that impractical, it's unlikely to be used. Instead, think about recording a brief meditation, or filming a quick lecture explicating your theme for the week. Here's where our emphasis on recycling themes comes in handy. It would be a lot of work to create new content each week keyed to a completely fresh theme. It's far easier—and just as impactful for students—to create one piece of content to share each month and have all your themes point back to this one idea. This doesn't need to have especially high production values. It could be as simple as going live on your social media and saving the recording to your profile.

It's wise to have an email newsletter list that your students can opt in to. (It may not be wise to mention this at studios with nonsolicitation policies in effect; see below.) Promising to send your playlist, quotes, a brief essay on the theme you used for class, or a preview of the next week's class incentivizes students to sign up for your newsletter. Depending on how much you enjoy writing, you could send whole series on the topics you discuss in class. This is both a way to share yoga's lessons and a way to establish your voice as a teacher. If you ask your readers to share your messages, and promote your newsletter on your social media, it can also expand your reach beyond your geographical market. This comes in really handy when you lead online classes or travel retreats. Note that it's wiser to focus on building an email newsletter than amassing large follower counts on social media platforms. You can move your newsletter platform from host to host; it belongs to you. Your followers are tied to a particular social media platform, and generally can't be moved to another.

Nonsolicitation Policies

If you rent space, lead outdoor classes, or run your own virtual studio, the takeaways you create and share can become an important feature of your teaching brand. If you teach at a studio run by someone else, check with your studio manager to see what their nonsolicitation policy is before distributing materials to your students. Otherwise, you risk garnering some serious ill will if you overstep your bounds. Some places will not share students' contact information, nor do they want teachers mentioning their newsletters or virtual offerings in class. Others don't mind. Sage's studio, Carolina Yoga, has a clear nonsolicitation policy in effect. The sentiment beyond the policy is to keep the studio brand clear and to prevent teachers actively promoting their external offerings on studio grounds— both physical and virtual. Sage encourages teachers to ask when they are unclear about what is acceptable and what isn't. It works out well for everyone involved. In the case of the lagniappes we've presented here, handing out paper with quotes would be fine; collecting newsletter sign-ups, or even mentioning a newsletter, would not. See Sage's 2020 book, *The Professional Yoga Teacher's Handbook,* for lots more on this.

Anything Else

Here, as in volume 1, we note resources or other thoughts and themes that could also connect. You might also like to use the space here to add your own notes on further reading you could suggest to your students, a different way to approach the theme, or even use this space to make a note of how well you think the theme lands the first time you teach it.

ADAPT AWAY

These themes are meant to be open to adaptation. We encourage you to make them your own by tweaking as needed. Here are some ways you can start:

Stick with a Theme for More Than One Class

If you teach various classes in a week, carry the same theme through each. Notice how the theme changes in different class formats. Good themes can apply to a wide range of classes, from very gentle to power flow. For example, the theme "Effort and Ease," in chapter 6, directly references the sutra *sthira sukham asanam* ("the pose should be steady and comfortable"). This can work in any class format, from the very strong to the very gentle, from heated power flow to restorative yoga with a sound bath. You could carry this theme with you over each of your classes in a week while saying different things about it every time.

Notice too how a theme naturally evolves each time you revisit it, the same way that your personal stories shift in meaning and your understanding of philosophical concepts crystallizes over time. Remember: It's OK to repeat your stories over and over. Your telling will vary from class to class, as will your student population. And no one will resent hearing a story retold—they may not even remember hearing it previously, and if they did, they'll remember it differently. Repetition is reassuring.

Make Your Own Themes

We want you to create more themes of your own! You'll find a few empty templates in this book to start now. You can also visit https://teachingyogabeyondtheposes .com and download our template in your favorite format. Then tweak it! You can change out headers, add space for your sequence notes, or do whatever works for your unique teaching style.

We also encourage you to continue with self-study. This can take various formats:

- **Explore** the resources we offer both in individual themes and at the start of every chapter. They will generate a host of ideas that you can build out over time.

- **Attend,** in person and online, a wide range of classes with a variety of teachers.

- **Notice** how teachers theme their classes, mimicking what works, and avoiding what you feel doesn't work. When you hear a phrase you love, jot it down!

- **Complete** our online course on theming—we will offer you direct mentorship! It's at https://teachingyogabeyondtheposes.com. We *love* getting to work with you one-on-one.

- **Share** and collaborate with us, both in that course and by tagging and messaging us (#teachingyogabeyondtheposes, contact info at https://teachingyogabeyondtheposes.com).

- **Share** and collaborate with other teachers! Start a theming group at your studio, or form one with your yoga teacher training cohort. Pass your themes around on paper or in a shared folder.

- **Read** ancient yogic texts. Read about the history of yoga. Read poetry. Read authors that inspire you and fill your well. Read and absorb.

- **Write!** Journal, keep a gratitude list, regularly think through your goals and your *sankalpa*. Be reflective in a spirit of self-compassion, self-acceptance, and serious inquiry. Get to know yourself well, and the themes that matter most to you will arise authentically.

We hope you will revel in the recognition that creating good themes is an exercise in mindful self-reflection and self-study. These are among the most important aspects of yoga! They will help you know yourself more and better, and by sharing them with your students, they will know themselves more and better. And by doing so, you'll be moving yourself, your students, and the world one step closer to liberation.

3

HOW YOU CAN BEST HELP YOUR STUDENTS

Students like authentic teachers offering simple, personally resonant, yet profound lessons. Offering these lessons and bits of philosophy isn't fluff or filling; it's part of the job we take on when we become yoga teachers. We offer messages as a way to connect to our students. We offer them as a way to connect students to ancient wisdom and philosophical ideas. We offer them as a way to connect our students to themselves. All of this connection is yoga.

In order to spread yoga, you need a student base. Even if it's just a small group of hard-core regulars you teach once a week, by sharing yoga's message with people, you are helping them move toward freedom and liberation, *moksha*. Let's look at how you can attract these students and, once you're connected with them, how you can help them best.

HOW THEMING CAN BUILD YOUR FOLLOWING

While we know you teach because you love yoga and you know it does profound good for your students, we know it feels good when your classes are fuller. So much outside you determines whether students attend: the day and time of the class, the season, the weather, and so on. But students also attend classes with teachers they love and enjoy. They come back to classes for many reasons, and one is that the ideas on offer strike a chord in them. In this way, good and thoughtful theming, like all the other parts of the class, will help you grow your student base.

Students come back when they relate to your messages. We don't typically get much feedback as yoga teachers—certainly not from the students. Usually the most verbal feedback you'll get is, "Thanks, that was a great class." The best positive feedback we have is returning students. They may not tell you exactly what they came back for, but we wager it's about how they felt during and after your class. It's not just about your creative choreography or skillful sequencing—in fact, that probably matters far less than you think, so don't feel like you need to plan out every second of class or come up with something creative and new every time. It's probably not the playlist you labored over, editing and adding songs like a consummate DJ. What matters most to students is how what you said and led in class made them feel. Remember the wonderful quote frequently attributed to Maya Angelou (but which most certainly predates her): "People will forget what you said, people will forget what you did, but people will never forget how you made them feel." This definitely applies in yoga class.

Do you give assists in your yoga classes? Or even offer something simple and special during Savasana, like a gentle shoulder press, or a little lavender-oil scalp massage? If so, you know that students come to expect and anticipate this part of class. They see it as a special treat, and they associate it with your specific classes and teaching style. In this same way, when you offer themes that allow your students to know themselves more, make them feel less alone and more connected to human experience, encourage them to reflect on their values, or help them regulate their challenging emotions, they start to expect that as part of the offering in your class, and they come back for your next message.

We discussed this briefly in chapter 2, but offering students some sort of takeaway is one way to grow the impact of your theme or message. If you have an email list for your classes and send newsletters to your students, you can further strengthen and reiterate your themes by writing them out. And you can do this *before* class, as a way to entice students to the practice or whet their appetites for the theme you'll be sharing. Alexandra teaches an all-levels community class in a small village west of where she lives. She's been teaching some version of the class for close to fifteen years, and some of the students have been attending for that long. Each week before class, she sends out an email that usually includes a little story from her life that week, along with how yoga or yoga philosophy or some other moral or spiritual lesson has given her a new way to look at the story she's sharing. In this way, students know what idea will be showing up in the practice. During class, the offered theme builds on what was already offered in the email. Students chat and joke with her and each other before class about the content of the email, and it grows the community and connection of the class. In this way, Alexandra spreads the message before, during, and after class.

FINDING THE STUDENTS WHO NEED YOUR MESSAGE

Any yoga class can be themed, no matter the format. But it's smart to be sure that the class style, the student population, and the message you deliver all work together harmoniously. Take some time to consider your students' expectations coming into the class. You could ask yourself (and your students, when you arrive!):

- How did they hear about this class? Was it from an internet search, a friend, a Groupon special? Will this source have primed them to receive philosophy along with movement in class?

- What is the title and, if relevant, the description of the class your students will have read? How does that set their expectations of what the class will be like, and what your message might be?

- Consider too that the time of day and the length of the class should impact the message you choose to offer and how you offer it. Night classes may feel more magical, and students attending at night might feel more open to spiritual ideas. Sunday morning classes may correlate with your students' childhood memories of church, and they may unconsciously seek and expect a dharma talk during that time. A midweek lunch-break class may be a better place for a pragmatic philosophical lesson. Meet your students where they're at.

- For returning students, what message have you been sharing lately? What related themes would be relevant to build on that?

- How much experience do these students have with yoga asana? With yoga philosophy? What is their comfort level with Sanskrit, with chanting?

- Given your students' experience and expectations, can you find a good fit between the theme you choose and the amount of other talking you'll be doing to cue the movement portions of class? Will you still be able to offer silence?

- Is there some timely local or global event that ties in to your theme?

Students who need your message may be very much like you or very much different from you. Don't presume that your message is falling flat just because the audience is dissimilar to you—or because they aren't smiling and nodding as you deliver it. Often a listening face reads like a bored or disaffected face. The sooner you can divorce your interpretation of a facial expression from your belief that what you're saying matters, the better a teacher you'll be.

FINDING THE RIGHT WORDS FOR YOUR STUDENTS

The words you choose to convey a theme may be more ephemeral and esoteric or more grounded and pragmatic, based on who's in the yoga room with you. Maybe your theme incorporates slang or swear words, depending on how well you know your students and what you think they'll hear best. Let your theming be a constant practice of creative reframing. Try a theme from a variety of angles, varying your sentences until you find language that rings true from your mouth and thus in your students' ears.

Remember, repetition is fine—and even more than that, it's necessary. We talked about this in volume 1 of *Teaching Yoga Beyond the Poses*. You're the only one who's ever heard every word to come out of your own mouth; students hear only about a third of the things you say. Never be concerned you're repeating yourself too much. You rarely are.

When in doubt, speak plainly and simplify. Bring your message back to its essential point. Or say less. In class, your voice is the only voice. It's your obligation to speak during class, but that also means that any silence in the room is yours to offer too. Use that power smartly and wisely. Give your students enough to listen to. Offer your students enough space to hear themselves.

Finally, recognize that the time on either side of the yoga practice is the best time to listen to your students. Greet them, make eye contact, and ask them questions. Speak during the practice; listen before and after.

·········· THE BASICS OF STORYTELLING ··········

Humans love stories. Good storytelling is the foundation of everything from education to gossip to sales copy writing. A story works best when it has memorable details, a surprising element, and a clear resolution. The memorable details include a relatable main character—that might be you, or it could be "a friend" (who's really you), or a real friend or family member. It could even be a public figure whom you heard interviewed or read some news about. Look to find some way for your students to connect to this main character. What do they want from life? How are they like the students? Or, if they are drastically different from your students, what other point of connection do they have? Around this relatable main character, sketch in other memorable details, like where and when the story takes place, so the scene is set for action.

The action of your story will captivate your audience when it has a surprising element. To find that and exploit it, consider what your listeners will expect to happen, then subvert those expectations. If Alexandra were telling her "No Blond Mommies" story that appears later in this book, she might say, "Heading home from the salon, I felt like a million bucks. I looked like a Disney princess. So, of course, I thought my daughter would be delighted to see my new hairstyle." This sets up the expectation that is then subverted when her daughter recoils and hides behind her bedroom door, freshly hung with a sign reading "No Blond Mommies." This plot twist keeps the listeners hooked—even in a short narrative that takes less than thirty seconds to recount.

Finally, the story you tell should have a clear resolution. The finale of your story should justify it being told, with some message or takeaway that ties right back to your theme. And to implicitly add "The End" to your personal story, you can pivot back to your theme using a quote, a few words about how this applies to the practice, or an invitation to your students to consider (and to share, if your class is small and conversational) how this story relates to their own personal experience.

Be human, and don't be afraid to be humorous too! Humor is OK when sharing a story in a yoga class. We don't always have to hold a sacred, ascetic space. But also don't be alarmed if no one laughs! And be aware of when you are using humor as a way to feel validated by your students. You are there to give to them; they are not there to give to you. Blank expressions are often a sign of deep inner work. Smiles and engagement might indicate a more superficial experience, which might be fine in some formats, but which in yoga doesn't allow time for the profound connection we seek.

As you tell your story in class, connecting your theme to both a personal and a universal experience, you must find the balance between making the theme relatable and making it all about you. As our evolved template now includes, we suggest that after you first present your message, you then give students a moment to look back and reflect about a time in their lives when this theme would have applied. And again at the end of class, ask students to think forward toward how this message will play out for them in the future. This can also become a prompt for journaling in your takeaway at the end of class. Adding in this time lets the students process your message more fully, and it centers their connection to your message, rather than your own experience.

PART 2

FRESH
THEMES

4

YOGA SUTRAS APPLICABLE TO MODERN LIFE

In the twenty-first-century West, we generally use Patanjali's Yoga Sutras as our touchtone scripture—it's the main, if not the only, one taught in yoga teacher trainings. But let's recognize that the Yoga Sutras is only one of the texts that references yoga, and it has extremely limited reference to asana. Much of the content of the later books of the text are focused on describing supernatural powers, so depending on your viewpoint, it may not be the canonical guide you think it is. It certainly is opaque and can be difficult to understand.

Still, there is much in the sutras that is worth studying and exploring. In this chapter, we present some of our favorite themes based on the sutras.

FOR MORE

More Themes to Explore

In the first volume of *Teaching Yoga Beyond the Poses,* you'll find several themes that reference the sutras, including one on each of the *yamas, niyamas,* and *kleshas; sthira* and *sukha, abhyasa* and *vairagya, samskara,* and the sutras' opening word, *atha.*

Reading on the Yoga Sutras

We love T. K. V. Desikachar's explication of the sutras in his book *The Heart of Yoga: Developing a Personal Practice* (Rochester, VT: Inner Traditions International, 1995).

The translation by Swami Satchidananda is a classic take on *The Yoga Sutras of Patanjali* (Yogaville, VA: Integral Yoga, 2012).

For applicability of how we may look at the Yoga Sutras from a modern lens, we like Nischala Joy Devi's *The Secret Power of Yoga: A Woman's Guide to the Heart and Spirit of the Yoga Sutras* (New York: Random House, 2007).

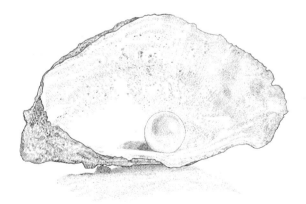

UNNECESSARY SUFFERING IS . . . UNNECESSARY

Expound on Your Theme and Connect It to a Personal and a Universal Experience

Sutra 2.16 is *"heyam duhkam anagatam,"* and in the well-known Satchidananda translation of this wisdom, this line is "Pain that has not yet come is avoidable." This sutra has to be considered in context: It follows sutras about the obstacles to joy and enlightenment (the kleshas), and it follows sutras that argue that, as the architects of our own lives, we are the ones most in the seat of our own divine understanding. Given that role, we can't avoid *all* suffering, but we can avoid the suffering that is internally derived.

The lesson of this sutra is similar to the Buddhist parable of the two arrows: The first arrow is the pain inflicted by an event or circumstance beyond your control. Imagine, for instance, that you offer a bright, cheery "Good morning" to a coworker who ignores you in response. That's the first arrow. Being ignored hurts! The second arrow can sometimes be a greater source of suffering, though. The second arrow is how you *respond* to the initial arrow. If you feel angry at your coworker, you're creating your own suffering. If you feel anxious that you did something to upset or offend your coworker, you're creating your own suffering. The pain of your coworker ignoring your kindness is unavoidable. But the pain that has not yet come—the pain of that second arrow—can be staved off through self-awareness, reflection, and a recognition that someone's response is not your burden to carry.

Chants, Quotes, Mantras, Poems, or Songs That Connect

Song: "An Ending, a Beginning" by Dustin O'Halloran

Quote: "Turn your wounds into wisdom." —Oprah Winfrey

Practices That Work with Your Theme

Balance exploration offers an opportunity to be challenged, to succeed or fail, and then to chart your own response to that success or failure. You could create a balance practice that gets progressively more challenging until everyone inevitably fails—and share that that's the point.

Distill Your Theme to a Short Sentence or Intention

What suffering can you opt out of?

Phrases or Sentences to Employ in These Parts of Your Class

OPENING	DURING MOVEMENTS
As we move today, you may feel a variety of things. Joy, freedom, and lightness are what I most hope you feel. But as we play with poses, you may find some movements that your body does not enjoy. When that happens, you get to notice your response and perhaps temper that response so that you opt out of avoidable suffering.	Is there avoidable suffering here? As we move on from that balance play, can you recognize that you didn't choose today's sequence, but you get to choose your response to it?
DURING PAUSES	**CLOSING**
In these moments of stillness and quiet, observe your mind. Are there any second arrows piercing your peace?	You cannot control external sources of pain and hurt. But you have the wisdom to lean away from unnecessary suffering.

Takeaway Ideas

If you share the Buddhist parable about the two arrows, a fun offering would be arrow-shaped bookmarks, maybe with Sutra 2.16 or a quote of your choice.

Anything Else

Students feel less alone when they hear that their trusted teacher also struggles with unnecessary suffering, so consider sharing a personal story that illustrates this in your own life.

Existential Kink by Carolyn Elliott* posits that we allow certain negative situations in our lives to continue because, in some perverse way, we enjoy the suffering they create. If you offered a series of themes on the topic of unnecessary suffering, you could also bring in this idea.

---

* Carolyn Elliott, *Existential Kink: Unmask Your Shadow and Embrace Your Power* (Newburyport, MA: Weiser Books, 2020).

TRANSCEND THE MIND TO FEEL THE DIVINE

Expound on Your Theme and Connect It to a Personal and a Universal Experience

The wisdom of divinity is like a radio station that's hard to adjust perfectly. We know it's there, and sometimes we catch momentary melodies of its beautiful music as we turn through the channels. Sometimes it's staticky. At other times it's so faint that we wonder if we're hearing a different song, seeping over from some other radio show.

Sutras 1.48 and 1.49 (*ritambhara tatra prajna,* "transcend the mind to feel the divine") offer us a reminder that our greatest truth is not learned from books. It's not garnered from experience. It's not the sum of the life we've lived so far. Rather, the truth of everything resides deep in ourselves. This divine intuition is always inside us, but it may take the right circumstances of yoga, meditation, and self-study to tune in to it, to find a moment where the station comes in clearly.

Embodied wisdom is something you've felt before. Imagine a time when an answer came so clearly that it didn't arrive from your mind. Or consider moments where you've felt so in sync with the currents and rhythms around you that you've barely felt separate from them. In these moments, you didn't create this wisdom through force or education or deep thinking; you simply arrived at a place where you could fully embody the wisdom that exists inside you, outside you, before you, and after you.

Chants, Quotes, Mantras, Poems, or Songs That Connect

Song: "Faith's Hymn" by Beautiful Chorus

Song: "Explorers of Infinity" by Marti Nikko and DJ Drez

Practices That Work with Your Theme

Focused pranayama like *dirga swasam* (three-part breath) or *sama vritti* (boxed breathing) can be a fun way to quietly lead students to their own divine internal wisdom. Both breathing practices may be led while students are seated or lying down.

Distill Your Theme to a Short Sentence or Intention

Your divine wisdom is beyond what you've read or what you've learned. It is not in your head or even your heart. It moves through you deeper and surer than simple intuition.

Phrases or Sentences to Employ in These Parts of Your Class

OPENING	DURING MOVEMENTS
As we move today, you get a chance to move without thinking. You get a chance to be guided and allow your divine wisdom to flow without restraint. Listen as we move.	We sometimes imagine that in silence, our wisdom bubbles magically to the surface. But sometimes movement and effort bring us into a space to truly hear.
DURING PAUSES	CLOSING
Return to your breath; maybe the breath practice we started with today. Tune in to the radio station of your divine wisdom.	As you move off your mat, do so with a renewed sense of your own divine wisdom.

Takeaway Ideas

Any little lagniappe that evokes spirituality is lovely here: a beautiful stone, for instance, gives your students a tangible reminder of their connection to the infinite.

Anything Else

It can be helpful to reassure students that in yoga we don't have a specific defined sense of divinity that is adhered to. If they come into class with their own faith tradition firmly in their mind, this lesson is like a translucent piece of parchment that lies on top—their religious story is still there, but the spiritual practice of yoga makes it shine beautifully and perhaps in a new way.

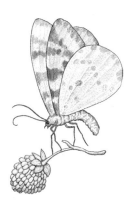

SUPREME DIVINITY

Expound on Your Theme and Connect It to a Personal and a Universal Experience

Sutra 1.24 tells us that the natural state of the divine in the universe is to be unbothered *(purushaviseshah isvarah)*. The divine, explains Patanjali, does not get caught up in desires, aversions, or what becomes of actions. Divinity simply is.

One understanding of divinity in yoga is that in the spirituality of yoga, divinity is not a force *outside* creation, but instead creation and creator are one. In this understanding of yoga, yoga is nondualist. (For much of classical yoga, however, it was a dualist spiritual philosophy—one of our favorite aspects of yoga is that it evolves, shifts, and changes.) In the nondualist view of yoga, to exist is to be a spiritual being. To exist is to be divine. And if divinity simply *is*, without all the attachments, stickiness, and hooks that humans spend our lives getting freed from, then we have a model for how we may move toward greater freedom: We can be more unbothered.

Chants, Quotes, Mantras, Poems, or Songs That Connect

Poem: "Buddha in Glory" by Rainer Maria Rilke

Song: "Within Me Is Boundless Love" by Beautiful Chorus

Practices That Work with Your Theme

Practice *anjali mudra* (prayer hands) in standing poses throughout class. Have students pause to connect to the divinity within them.

Include simple repetitive movements or kriya sequences that give students a chance to shake off their bothers.

Distill Your Theme to a Short Sentence or Intention

Embody your own divinity by being unbothered.

Phrases or Sentences to Employ in These Parts of Your Class

OPENING	DURING MOVEMENTS
Did you come into class today bothered? Now that you're here, can you start to cultivate freedom from your bothers?	How can you be more unbothered here? How can you be more spacious, more free, more divine as you flow?
DURING PAUSES	**CLOSING**
Notice, as you rest, how this is all there is: no bothers. Just your breath, just your body.	Move into the world in a way that is unbothered. Grant others the freedom of your ease.

Takeaway Ideas

At the start of class, place a penny or a small object at the top of students' mats. At some point, identify it as a tangible representation of their bothers. Invite them to give it away or toss it away after they leave class.

Anything Else

The Buddhist concept of *shenpa,* elucidated often by author Pema Chödrön, helps us see that when we experience a "hook" (like an annoyance or a bother) we often shut down and turn away—from others, from ourselves, from our own divinity. This is a concept you might dive into further.

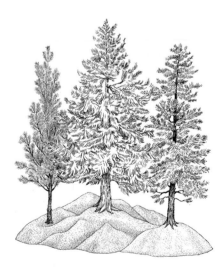

HISTORY CAN DISTRACT

Expound on Your Theme and Connect It to a Personal and a Universal Experience

Sutra 4.27 is *pratyayantarani samskarebhyah*. These words imply that past beliefs or impressions can still affect your mind, even if you have moved higher up the spiral staircase of your enlightenment. Essentially, if you allow it to, the past—and its experiences, beliefs, and stories—can distract you from the present.

This may seem lofty at first, but it's deeply relatable. Have you ever shared a challenging story from your past and noticed that you still feel the emotional effects of it? You may be in the midst of opening up to a new friend, and suddenly you find yourself flushed with anger about a long-ago injustice. Or perhaps you've been mid-daydream when you suddenly noticed that you were thinking up cutting retorts that a past version of you would have employed in a long-dormant argument. Sometimes we need to reprocess emotions of anger, frustration, pain, or hurt. You may need to do this with a trusted spouse, friend, or therapist as part of your healing journey. But sometimes you can also get stuck in an emotional loop, recycling past impressions that no longer need affect you in the present. This is an example of how history can seep into the present moment and pull you from a space of calm, a space of awareness, a space of intentionality, and a space of peace. History, if you let it, can distract you.

Chants, Quotes, Mantras, Poems, or Songs That Connect

Song: "Be Here Now" by Mason Jennings

Poem: "It Was Like This: You Were Happy" by Jane Hirshfield

Quote: "Forget everything else. Keep hold of this alone and remember it: Each of us lives only now, this brief instant. The rest has been lived already, or is impossible to see." —Marcus Aurelius, *Meditations*, translated by Gregory Hays

Practices That Work with Your Theme

Have students practice *sitali pranayama* (cooling breath) and share how it can be used as a practice for cooling down challenging emotions.

Choose a challenging pose, perhaps Revolved Triangle Pose, and revisit it several times in the practice. Each time, invite students to come to the pose fresh, without carrying in their impressions of their last exploration of it.

Distill Your Theme to a Short Sentence or Intention

The stories of your life can pull you out of the moment. Stay present.

Phrases or Sentences to Employ in These Parts of Your Class

OPENING	DURING MOVEMENTS
Notice how you've arrived here today: Check in with your emotional state and where your mind is. Are you fully present? If you notice you are reviewing any past events or happenings of your day, connect to your breathing until your mind is fully present in the now.	You've seen this pose before; we've explored it already this practice. Can you come into this shape without any impressions or assumptions from your previous play here?
DURING PAUSES	**CLOSING**
(Allow there to be silence for a bit before you speak.) Where does your mind go in this quietness? Do you stay fully in the room, or are you revisiting another experience or moment? Does your history distract you here?	The stories of your life, your challenges, are great gifts and lessons. They can help you be more discerning and aware in the present. But they can also distract you from the present if you get caught up in the injustices or frustrations of the past. The present is all we have.

Takeaway Ideas

Offer each student a scrap of paper and invite them to write down a snippet of history that disrupts their present. Gather up these scraps and promise not to read them and ceremonially destroy them after class.

Anything Else

This theme is a powerful one, but it can be preachy if you don't pair it with something personal and maybe even lighthearted. Consider sharing a story from your own life about a time some past event stole a little bit of your peace in the present.

SEE THE FOREST, NOT THE TREES

Expound on Your Theme and Connect It to a Personal and a Universal Experience

In Sutra 2.47, Patanjali is offering the age-old reminder: Just chill. Sometimes your effort—whether in asana, in your own spiritual growth, or in anything—can be an impediment to your success. The force you exert in pursuit of some achievement in yoga can become the obstacle. *Prayatna saithilya ananta samapattibhyam* tells us that when we back off from extreme efforts, we can often more easily find our connection with divinity—the larger purpose of the practice.

Another way to think about this is that on the path of yoga, you can get stuck in the trees: the details of how to do a breathing practice or the need to master a certain pose, for instance. The forest is the bigger picture, the reminder that the point and purpose of yoga is to unite you with your own essential nature. And that will happen whether you pretzel yourself into Scorpion Pose or not. It will happen if alternate-nostril breathing makes you cough. It will happen if you find yourself distracted during every meditation practice. It will happen as you remain steadfast—but not tense with the effort of that steadfastness.

Chants, Quotes, Mantras, Poems, or Songs That Connect

Song: "Ocean" by dontask

Song: "Roll with Me" by Davie

Quote: "Practice and all is coming." —K. Pattabhi Jois

Practices That Work with Your Theme

Any practices that are not rigid and encourage letting go. You may try to offer free-flowing movements during part of class. Or lead students through a familiar sequence, like a round or two of Sun Salutations—and then invite them to move through the same sequence on their own with no need to get each step or pose "right."

Distill Your Theme to a Short Sentence or Intention

Is your effort or rigidity holding you back from true connection to yourself?

Phrases or Sentences to Employ in These Parts of Your Class

OPENING	DURING MOVEMENTS
Sometimes we arrive in class, treating it like one more accomplishment, one more box to check off on the journey toward better health or more mindfulness. We may imagine that we have to do *something* to make that happen: practice in some specific way, or feel deeply grounded in Savasana, or something else that signifies we have "achieved" what we set out to. If that resonates with you, I invite you to soften. Relax. Notice you have arrived in yoga, and that is enough.	Where can you relax more into this shape? Where can you relinquish force?
DURING PAUSES	**CLOSING**
There is no effort required here. Can you recognize this space of effortless existence as yoga?	Have faith that your practice is moving you toward greater self-knowledge and liberation—whatever your experience of your yoga practice tonight was!

Takeaway Ideas

Since the essential message here is "Have faith and let go," it would be a fun idea to build a playlist based on that theme. You could play it in class or not, but either way, you could share the playlist with your students so they can keep this theme alive while they jam out on the way home.

Anything Else

If this theme seems like familiar territory to you, keep in mind that it may not feel that way to your students. We often joke that all themes really boil down to just a few essential messages. Any message that helps your students "be present" and "let go" is a good one.

DEDICATION AND DETACHMENT

Expound on Your Theme and Connect It to a Personal and a Universal Experience

In earlier sutras, Patanjali spells out that true yoga is the cessation of the mind's fluctuations. In Sutra 1.12, *abyhasa vairagyabhyam tannirodha,* we begin to understand how: through dedication and detachment.

The true benefits of yoga don't arrive quickly. When you're new to the practice, there is a lot of fun to be had in challenging poses, transportive class experiences of music and low lighting, lavender-scented Savasana assists, and the glimmer of something else that peeks out behind and between all of this. It's that something else—that reminder of divinity, that awareness of prana, that experience of kundalini rising—that yoga practitioners notice and get curious about. We practice to find those mystical moments, and then the practice transforms as we realize those moments are not outside us, not something we can chase and pin down, but they arise from within ourselves and are omnipresent, if sometimes hard to access. We practice to connect more deeply, to allow our awareness of that "something else" to grow fuller. We practice with consistent effort and dedication. And the more dedicated we are, the more we arrive.

At the same time, we must move through life—and through our dedication to yoga—with some amount of dispassion. If we are overly invested in some particular experience or outcome, we grip too deeply, and we hold on too tightly.

Instead, if we sit with the definition of yoga as something akin to "stopping the mind's chaos," we recognize that our minds are most chaotic when we feel strong emotions. Patanjali suggests that because of this, detachment is necessary. Consider that you know from experience that when your emotional life is calmer, and when you feel more stable in your feelings, you walk in the world clearer and with fewer misperceptions.

The path of yoga requires dedication and dispassion in equal measure.

Chants, Quotes, Mantras, Poems, or Songs That Connect

Song: "Worried Mind" by Megafaun

Song: "I" by Benn Jordan

Practices That Work with Your Theme

If you're comfortable offering *nadi shodhana* (alternate-nostril breathing), that connects beautifully to emotional equanimity.

Distill Your Theme to a Short Sentence or Intention

Can you feel dedicated and present in today's practice without grasping?

Phrases or Sentences to Employ in These Parts of Your Class

OPENING	DURING MOVEMENTS
We love the idea of balancing dispassion and dedication. Like so many of the physical poses in yoga, this ask is very much a paradox. Somewhere between deep dedication and attachment, there is a hair's breadth emotional state where we can be both fully present and dedicated, yet also unaffected by the happenings around us or the outcome of our dedication. That's what we're looking for today. That little space.	Are you fully here and dedicated to this movement? Can you be here fully without attaching to any specific way that this pose has to be?
DURING PAUSES	**CLOSING**
In this moment of rest, let go of the dedication. You are here. That is enough. There is nothing more to do right now.	Dedication and dispassion aren't messages just for a physical asana practice. This is a mantra that can guide your life: your partnerships and relationships, the way you approach work. Before you leave this space, consider spaces in your life that may benefit from this approach.

Takeaway Ideas

Gifts that fade beautifully represent dedication and dispassion. A small flower, if it's seasonally appropriate, can offer your students the message of dedication (consider how much work it was for this flower to bloom!) and dispassion (and yet, its bloom will fade).

Anything Else

You might point out to your students that the message of this sutra is similar to a major theme from the Bhagavad Gita: Do your work with no attachment to outcome. We offered a theme on that idea in volume 1 of *Teaching Yoga Beyond the Poses*.

5

OM SHANTI AND
OTHER YOGIC THOUGHT

Beyond the sutras, there are some common yoga terms that deserve being presented in class. Leading themes on these words and ideas is a way to bring newer students up to speed on some things they'll hear in class—and to contextualize the phrases that often have been maladapted and wedged into the context of Western movement classes.

FOR MORE

More Themes to Explore

Lokah samastha sukino bhavantu: May all beings everywhere be happy and free.

"Hare Krishna"

Spanda: the radiant energy of creation

Lila: the play of the divine

Moksha: liberation

Reading

Susanna Barkataki's "How to Decolonize Your Yoga Practice" (www.susanna barkataki.com/post/how-to-decolonize-your-yoga-practice) offers a lot of thoughtful ways to consider yoga as Western practitioners.

For a scholarly deeper dive into yoga philosophy, we like *Roots of Yoga,* edited by James Mallinson and Mark Singleton (New York: Penguin, 2017).

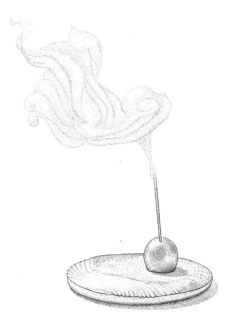

CHANGE IS THE NATURAL STATE

Expound on Your Theme and Connect It to a Personal and a Universal Experience

Parinamavada is a cosmological concept that at its simplest says that constant change is the normal, expected nature of the universe. Constant change in your life, in your mind, in your mood is to be expected—indeed, it is the essence of everything. When you accept these constant fluctuations of the ocean of life, rather than resist the currents and ripples, you find it much easier to float along, riding the waves and not drowning in them. And as Greek philosopher Heraclitus said, you can never step in the same river twice, because everything is always in flux.

When Alexandra teaches on this, she often shares a personal story about her young daughter responding unhappily when Alexandra dyed her hair a new color. Her daughter was extremely unmoored by her mom having new hair and created a sign for her playroom door that read "No Blond Mommies!" Hilarious as that is, it also reminds us how resistant we can feel to any change, even when it doesn't affect us. Being blond didn't change Alexandra's parenting, for instance.

Yet despite the fact that change is inevitable and constant, we are still often surprised or angry when things change. Parinamavada tells us that change is the natural state of things, which allows us to recognize that we can have empathy for ourselves and for others when a response to change is frustration, fear, or anxiety.

Chants, Quotes, Mantras, Poems, or Songs That Connect

Song: "We Are Okay" by Joshua Radin

Quote: "There is nothing bad in undergoing change—or good in emerging from it." —Marcus Aurelius, *Meditations,* translated by Gregory Hays

Chant: Repetition of a simple chant, like multiple rounds of Om

Mantra: I'm OK in the face of change.

Aphorism: Let go or be dragged.

Practices That Work with Your Theme

Practice balance poses and remind students as they balance to accept the inconsistency that arises—and embrace it. Or play with coming into familiar poses in new ways. Invite your students to explore change and how it makes them feel. If you think the challenge or newness may bring up frustration in students, as change can do, incorporate open-mouthed sighing in moments of stillness and rest.

Distill Your Theme to a Short Sentence or Intention

Change is the natural state. Once we internalize that truth, we will find more space to accept change rather than resist it. I'm OK in the face of change.

Phrases or Sentences to Employ in These Parts of Your Class

OPENING	DURING MOVEMENTS
Hearing "Change is inevitable" is much easier than *absorbing* "Change is inevitable." We can look to nature and the fluxes of our own lives to know that change is the natural state. But even though we understand that change is a constant, we spend much of our lives creating systems that keep things static and routine. In our practice today, you'll experience change—and lovingly notice your reaction to it.	How did it feel to move into that shape differently than you're used to? Did you feel resistance to that change? Can you validate those feelings and empathize with the part of you that always wants to know what's going to happen next?
DURING PAUSES	**CLOSING**
Even in stillness, change persists. Notice how your body is changed here from when you arrived today. Notice how the quality of your breath has changed.	As you move off your mat and into the world, you get a chance to model what we explored on the mat today. Perhaps there is a perspective shift, like more empathy for yourself, as you navigate the inevitability of change.

Takeaway Ideas

A little card that says "Let go or be dragged" or "I'm OK in the face of change" might be a nice reminder.

Anything Else

If you offer challenging balance poses or unfamiliar ways to transition into poses, you may also want to offer an extralong sweet Savasana, where you offer hands-on assists to help your students feel grounded by the end of class.

Brad Stulberg's book *Master of Change: How to Excel When Everything Is Changing—Including You* (New York: HarperOne, 2023) gives a useful perspective on the inevitability of change and ways to shift your relationship to change.

SAHAJA: ALREADY ENLIGHTENED

Expound on Your Theme and Connect It to a Personal and a Universal Experience

We both have backgrounds in English literature. One phrase that gained popularity—and grew overused—in critical academic writing during Sage's time in graduate school was "always already." This phrase resonates here: *sahaja* says you are always already enlightened. Sahaja is sometimes translated as "spontaneous," but the implication of the word is more akin to effortless, natural, or automatic than it is to the idea of, say, a rapidly made decision. Sahaja reminds you of your essential nature. The journey of yoga may be a long and circuitous one, but the beginning and ending are the same: It starts with you and ends with you. You have already arrived. You are always already enlightened. Yoga is just an opportunity to wake to that truth.

Chants, Quotes, Mantras, Poems, or Songs That Connect

Song: "I Am Light" by India.Arie

Song: "Drift" by Benji Lewis

Mantra: I know what I already know. I embody all that I am. I am whole.

Practices That Work with Your Theme

Allow students to explore in poses with spontaneous, intuitive movement. This may be something you explain at the start of the practice and then weave into the sequence.

Distill Your Theme to a Short Sentence or Intention

You are already enough.

Phrases or Sentences to Employ in These Parts of Your Class

OPENING	DURING MOVEMENTS
Coming into the practice, you are setting aside time to simply connect with what is already.	What if you already knew how to hold this shape with grace and calm? How would that feel? And can you access that grace and calm right now?
DURING PAUSES	**CLOSING**
As you rest, feel the peace that was always already inside.	Now we're getting ready to move off the mat and back into the world with other people. Can you make a commitment to see the enlightenment already present in people you interact with? Let's start by looking at each other in recognition.

Takeaway Ideas

One of the teachers at our studio offers, with studio permission, business cards printed with his theme for every class he teaches. Often the cards just have a word or a phrase, and of course his approved contact info: It's theming plus marketing. We love the idea of just offering students the word *sahaja* to serve as a reminder of this message.

Anything Else

Being reminded of our essential wholeness is a powerful message. This is a theme you may want to explore over a number of classes.

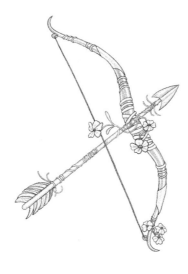

CHITTA VRITTI NIRODHA: FLUCTUATIONS OF THE MIND

Expound on Your Theme and Connect It to a Personal and a Universal Experience

The Yoga Sutras acknowledge up front—as early as the second sutra—that human nature means the mind is constantly in flux with a running commentary. This is reassuring—so many of us are alarmed to find there's a lot of mental noise when we sit for meditation. We think that means we're failing at it. On the contrary, it means we've managed to pay attention long enough to see things as they are. The work of meditation is then to keep coming back to this attention, instead of identifying with the fluctuations.

Once we do, we can start to let these fluctuations still and quiet. Then, as the next sutra tells us, we can rest in our true nature, as the seer of these thoughts and not as the thoughts themselves.

We know everyone experiences this. Ellen DeGeneres famously described being in yoga: "I'm looking out of my third eye and everything that I'm supposed to be doing. It's amazing what comes up when you sit in that silence. 'Mama keeps whites bright like the sunlight. Mama's got the magic of Clorox 2.'" You might have a similar surprise in store when you settle. What arises could be a mindless advertising jingle, it could be self-criticism, it could be the solution to a problem you've been chewing on. All of these are places your mind will take you. Just remember that the destination is not the point. It's noticing that your mind is churning, and abiding to let it settle.

Chants, Quotes, Mantras, Poems, or Songs That Connect

Song: "Where Is My Mind?" by Pixies

Aphorism: Don't believe everything you think.

Scripture: "Be still, and know that I am God" —Psalms 46:10

Practices That Work with Your Theme

A quiet hold of a pose with a few well-timed prompts to notice the mental experience as it unfolds.

Distill Your Theme to a Short Sentence or Intention

Let your mind grow quiet and be the seer.

Phrases or Sentences to Employ in These Parts of Your Class

OPENING	DURING MOVEMENTS
We'll have a little less talk from me than usual in this practice. This will give you time to observe the places your mind wants to go, both while we are moving and while we are still.	Notice how your mental chatter has changed during this flow.
DURING PAUSES	**CLOSING**
When you slow down, does your mind's running commentary ramp up? Or can you settle fully here into rest, both physical and mental?	Notice the state of your mental chatter now. If it's as loud as ever, know that that's human! If it's any quieter, could this be the new normal, a level-setting that you can carry with you off the mat?

Takeaway Ideas

A slip of paper with Sutra 1.2: "Yoga is the cessation of the fluctuations of the mind."

Anything Else

This is a great theme to offer over the course of several weeks. You could add in a meditation at the beginning or end of class, lengthening it by a minute or two each week, to give students more time to be the seer and stop identifying with the thoughts.

PRATIPAKSHA BHAVANA AND THE ANCIENT ART OF COGNITIVE REAPPRAISAL

Expound on Your Theme and Connect It to a Personal and a Universal Experience

Pratipaksha bhavana translates to something like "cultivating the opposite." It shows up in Yoga Sutra 2.33, but it's not just ancient wisdom; it's also a modern-day practice for the regulation of emotions called *cognitive reappraisal*. Cognitive reappraisal implores us to look at a situation from an alternative perspective.

One anecdote that Sage shared in *The Professional Yoga Teacher's Handbook* comes from Alexandra's teaching career: One time a student came to class, but shortly after class started, she got an unhappy look on her face and left. The story Alexandra told herself in the moment involved this student not liking the sequence, the playlist, or Alexandra! Pratipaksha bhavana would have allowed her to imagine a different perspective: What if the woman left because she felt physically unwell? What if she left because she just remembered an important phone call she had to make? What if she left because she suddenly became certain she left her stove on? If you remember this anecdote from Sage's book, you'll know that this was indeed the case, and the student rushed home just in time to find her teakettle empty and glowing red, but thankfully no other harm done.

Cognitive reappraisal reminds us not to assume the worst of other people. It reminds us that there may be a different reason for their actions than the initial one we surmise. Intentionally pushing ourselves to think past our first theory about someone's behavior, intention, or action can move us out of an emotional rut that's not serving us or anyone around us.

Chants, Quotes, Mantras, Poems, or Songs That Connect

Song: "You're Not Free" by Frazey Ford

Song "Samskara" by Little Symphony

Song: "Rainbow" by Kacey Musgraves

Practices That Work with Your Theme

You might ask students in advance what poses they think of as their nemesis poses and incorporate those in the practice so they can try to change their perspective on them.

Distill Your Theme to a Short Sentence or Intention

Can you move past your first assumption? Can you see this a different way?

Phrases or Sentences to Employ in These Parts of Your Class

OPENING	DURING MOVEMENTS
We're going to play with poses today that you've shared are challenging. Your exploration today will be to let go of the assumptions you already have about how these poses make you feel. What story do you tell yourself about your nemesis pose? Can you shift that?	Heading into this pose, what are your assumptions? What story do you want to tell yourself? What emotions are coming up?
DURING PAUSES	**CLOSING**
We've left this shape behind now. Did it feel different? Did approaching the pose, and your assumptions about it, with intention shift anything for you?	We do so much on the mat that is applicable in our daily lives. Let's take some time in silence now. Allow your mind to drift to a place in your life where there is a situation of discomfort. Is there another perspective you may be missing? Is there another way to see things?

Takeaway Ideas

A few printed-out journaling prompts that connect to this idea and allow students to continue to see the applicability to their daily lives could be powerful.

Anything Else

It's useful to remind students that sometimes we get stuck on a particular view of things because we don't share our thoughts, instead allowing our interpretation of something to exist only in our mind. The easiest way to consider alternative perspectives is to ask others for theirs.

OM SHANTI: PEACE

Expound on Your Theme and Connect It to a Personal and a Universal Experience

Peace is not a concept particular to any one culture or language. In yoga, we may associate peace with a clear mind, or with surrender to divinity, or with the recognition that there is no separation between ourselves and everything else. During our time on earth, we may cultivate moments of peace by way of being present in the moment and expressing gratitude for that moment. Peace offers great equanimity. We may argue that each begets the other, with no clear answer of what comes first: do we feel great mental composure and emotional calm because of peace, or is that what creates the feeling of peace? Regardless, since we know that when we welcome states of presence, calm, and focus, we feel peaceful, we can capitalize on that and do our best to create an environment that moves us toward greater peace.

Consider how hard it is to feel calm in a messy room. To feel truly grounded and peaceful, disarray may need to be tamed. The same is true of your mind: If there are competing goals, a thousand spinning plates in the air, and no time for rest and renewal, your mind is not going to be settled. A practice on *shanti* is a practice that emphasizes groundedness, composure, presence, and stillness. But it's also helpful to note that in today's very connected word, it's hard to find stillness and silence. Finding shanti may become a practice of finding peace amidst the chaos: letting the text chime be a reminder to stay present rather than a call to engage.

Chants, Quotes, Mantras, Poems, or Songs That Connect

Chant: *Om, shanti, shanti, shanti,* peace, peace, peace

Song: "Shanti" by Wah!

Poem: "Messenger" by Mary Oliver

Practices That Work with Your Theme

The breath practice of a physiological sigh is a lovely breath practice to cultivate calm and peace. This practice involves inhaling deeply through your nose and then pausing at the top. You then add a last little inhale, a little sip of breath through your nose, to completely fill your lungs. After another short pause, you sigh out through your mouth.

Distill Your Theme to a Short Sentence or Intention

Breathe in peace, breathe out chaos.

Phrases or Sentences to Employ in These Parts of Your Class

OPENING	DURING MOVEMENTS
Coming into class today, what's in disarray in your mind? Can you try taking some deep, full breaths? Can you remind yourself that you are no longer responding to emails, or actively parenting your children, or planning anything? You're just here. And for the next hour, your only job is to be present with yourself and your breath in service of your own peace.	Without getting obsessive about alignment, how can you clean up the lines of this shape to feel more at ease? As we flow through this movement again, notice how you've refined it every time. Do you feel the freedom and peace that come from smoothing out and better connecting breath with movement?
DURING PAUSES	**CLOSING**
Can you settle into the peace of this moment? It's an oasis within an oasis, a refuge within a refuge.	As you prepare to move back into the messy world, how can you carry a sense of centered peace with you? Is there a phrase or a feeling or a gesture, like this current one of your hand resting on your heart, that can bring you back to peace?

Takeaway Ideas

Equip students with a pen and paper before class and ask them to write down every synonym they can think of for the word *peace* to help develop an intention for the practice. The concept of shanti may resonate better with someone when they find their own language for it.

Anything Else

There are so many lovely books to recommend to students on this theme. *Peace Is Every Step: The Path of Mindfulness in Everyday Life* by Thich Nhat Hahn (New York: Random House, 1992) comes to mind.

NAMASTE: I BOW TO YOU

Expound on Your Theme and Connect It to a Personal and a Universal Experience

When yoga teachers in Western cultures end their yoga classes with "Namaste," the implied meaning is something like, "The light in me sees and honors the light in you," or "I bow to you." In India, the word *namaste* is used in greeting, mostly to elders or someone to whom respect is shown. It's not used as a good-bye, and it's not imbued with quite the same reverence we see at the end of yoga classes. For this reason, we have both moved away from using "Namaste" to end our classes. But the implied meaning—I see you fully, I acknowledge you, and I bow to you—is a beautiful one! You might share with your students how deeply you believe in that message, rather than using the inaccurate shorthand of "Namaste" to signal it. Indeed, we bet the meaning will land even more then, since most students probably don't really know what "Namaste" means, where it comes from, and what it has evolved to suggest in Western classes.

One crucial aspect of group movement classes, whether yoga or something more akin to boot camp, is that the students are showing up to be *seen*. Don't we all want to be seen? Who doesn't love when others notice their new clothes or haircut? In the role of the teacher, you have a unique power: You can notice others, and you can encourage them to see each other.

Chants, Quotes, Mantras, Poems, or Songs That Connect

Part of why people loved the movie *Avatar* was the Na'vi phrase, "I see you." In the imaginary language, it's *Oel ngati kameie*. This phrase points right to the heart of the metaphorical way we use "Namaste" in class (and we can use it without baggage or fear of appropriation).

Practices That Work with Your Theme

Consider setting up the room in rows facing in toward the center. This offers an opportunity for students to see each other—and literally to bow to each other if you are coming into standing or seated forward folds. Be sure to leave some spaces for those who want to opt out. This could be a second row of mats behind one of the front rows, or a space at each end that won't have another student directly across from it. Or artfully stagger the rows so that the eye contact is less direct but still present.

Distill Your Theme to a Short Sentence or Intention

See the light in yourself and others.

Phrases or Sentences to Employ in These Parts of Your Class

OPENING	DURING MOVEMENTS
Without staring at your classmates, use your peripheral vision to register that we are all here together to work on a common project: being present in the moment, by using the practice of yoga as a tool for focused awareness.	Again use your peripheral vision to recognize that other students are going through the same shapes and encountering the same challenges. Let the sound of your breath be a message to them: "I see you. We are in this together."
DURING PAUSES	**CLOSING**
Bow to yourself here. Bow to the practice here.	As you blink your eyes open, again see your classmates—your teammates—with your peripheral vision. If you feel comfortable, look around the room and make eye contact. We see each other, and this is a powerful way to recognize the power of practicing in community.

Takeaway Ideas

Share more with your students about the meaning and usage of the word *namaste*. Susanna Barkataki has plenty of resources online (www.susannabarkataki.com) as well as suggestions for alternatives teachers can use.

Anything Else

Two alternative words that work as both greeting and farewell: *Aloha* and *ciao*. Kripalu yogis often use the phrase *jai bhagwan,* which invokes divinity—it's sort of like "Praise God." It's a nice way to end or begin class.

6

SIMPLE AND PROFOUND

Sometimes the deepest lessons are also the simplest. The themes in this chapter might lend themselves especially well to beginner classes or classes in more secular settings, like a gym.

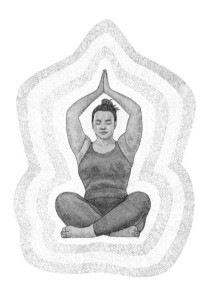

FOR MORE

More Themes to Explore

Consider theming around simple abstract words that we use in everyday life. There's a lot to say about the word *love*, for instance. It's simple, but you could theme on it a thousand different ways and introduce something new each time. Consider other simple and profound words: *joy, good, vulnerability, listen, hear,* and so on.

Reading

Keep your eyes open, because *everything* you read has the potential to inspire simple and profound themes. Children's books are especially potent, and they hit on a collective subconscious nerve. You could start with:

A. A. Milne, *Winnie-the-Pooh*

Antoine de Saint-Exupéry, *The Little Prince*

Charlie Mackesy, *The Boy, the Mole, the Fox and the Horse*

Margery Williams, *The Velveteen Rabbit*

Sandra Boynton, *Happy Hippo, Angry Duck*

Matt de la Peña and Christian Robinson, *Last Stop on Market Street*

Aaron Blabey, *Thelma the Unicorn*

Cori Doerrfeld, *The Rabbit Listened*

Carter Goodrich, *Nobody Hugs a Cactus*

Jon J. Muth, *Zen Shorts*

BE HERE NOW

Expound on Your Theme and Connect It to a Personal and a Universal Experience

There are probably a million ways to theme on the concept of presence, and we encourage you to find as many of them as you can. "Be here now" is a call to arrive in the present. It is a gentle command to fully show up in the moment of *now*, which is the only moment that really exists.

Now is, in fact, the first word of the Yoga Sutras. What better reminder that now is of primary importance! It is the moment in which we breathe, in which we hold agency, in which we can hone our presence through the practice of yoga.

Chants, Quotes, Mantras, Poems, or Songs That Connect

Song: "Be Here Now" by Beautiful Chorus

Quote: "How we spend our days is, of course, how we spend our lives. What we do with this hour, and that one, is what we are doing." —Annie Dillard

Poem: "Days" by Philip Larkin

Practices That Work with Your Theme

The entirety of yoga! As the teacher, you can continually cue students to come back to now. A check-in using the senses can help (see "During Movements" and "During Pauses" below).

Distill Your Theme to a Short Sentence or Intention

This is it.

Phrases or Sentences to Employ in These Parts of Your Class

OPENING	DURING MOVEMENTS
Take a moment to recognize what it took to get here. You might have left work early, hired a sitter, or fought through traffic in order to be here. You might have overcome your self-consciousness or done work to revise your own self-image to step onto your mat. What better way can you honor the work you've already put in than being fully present here and now?	As we move, can you use your senses to stay present? What do you see now? What do you hear now? What do you feel now?
DURING PAUSES	**CLOSING**
Again, be in this moment in this body. What do you see, even if your eyes are closed? What do you hear, even in the quiet? How does your breath feel?	As you prepare to move back into the rhythm of your life, what cue can you use to remind yourself to be here now?

Takeaway Ideas

So often, the best takeaway is the words themselves. Offer your students a little note card that says "Be here now."

Anything Else

It may be worth sharing a little about Ram Dass, who popularized this phrase, and his work on presence.

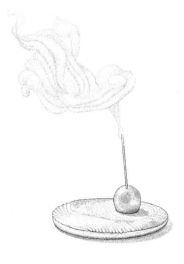

INHALE WHAT YOU NEED; EXHALE WHAT YOU DON'T

Expound on Your Theme and Connect It to a Personal and a Universal Experience

The idea of inhaling what you need and exhaling what you don't can sound reductive, and at its worst can fall back on "Let go of that which no longer serves you," which grates us with its implication that things are here to serve us—or suggests that we always have the power to immediately drop what we wish to. If that were the case, neither of us would ever wash a dish again because washing dishes most definitely doesn't "serve" us! But when you sit with this theme, it's also deeply powerful. That's in part because it is quite literally what happens with every breath. You take in what you need—oxygen—and release what you don't—carbon dioxide. Further, what you release with each exhale would ultimately kill you if you didn't let it go, and likewise you would expire if you didn't intake fresh oxygen regularly.

Even more, you can't breathe in and get what you need if you don't first breathe out to make room for the new. This is a lesson Sage learned as a swimmer, especially in open-water racing, where waves and water churned up by other swimmers might wind up in your mouth when you turn to breathe. You have to be completely ready for the new breath by letting go of the old. Otherwise, you won't get what you need in the limited time your head is out of the water.

While this cycle happens constantly with the breath, it also applies across a broad range of life experiences, from house decluttering to ending a relationship, losing a job, or growing on any level. Thus it's always a salient theme for class. Every student—every human!—is in the midst of constant change, breath to breath, pose to pose, day to day, year to year.

Chants, Quotes, Mantras, Poems, or Songs That Connect

Song: "Breathe" by Pink Floyd

Song: "Let It Go" by Essie Jain

Poem: "A Poem for Someone Who Is Juggling Her Life" by Rose Cook

Chant: Breathe it in; let it go

Practices That Work with Your Theme

All breath exercises! At the start of the practice, extended exhalations; at the end of the practice, extended inhalations.

Inhales that lift things, like your arms, and exhales that lower them.

Distill Your Theme to a Short Sentence or Intention

Out with the old, in with the new.

Take what you need; leave what you don't.

Phrases or Sentences to Employ in These Parts of Your Class

OPENING	DURING MOVEMENTS
What are you ready to set down and let go of in your practice today? When you let go of what you don't need, you're making room to pick up what you do need.	What are you picking up here? What are you taking on? How does this shape or movement bring in freshness?
DURING PAUSES	**CLOSING**
Open your mouth and exhale with a sigh: *ah-h-h*. Let go. Release what you don't need.	As we head into final relaxation, see if you can set everything down. Let it all go.
Is your mind holding on to something you could let go of?	As we prepare to move off the mat, what do you need to bring in?

Takeaway Ideas

A printed copy of the "Poem for Someone Who Is Juggling Her Life," or its closing line: "Let it all fall sometimes."

Instructions for a simple breath exercise, maybe playing with breath ratios.

Anything Else

Bring your humanity to this theme. Talk to your students about what you're working on "exhaling." They need to know you're also exhaling cranky kids or delayed emails or whatever is weighing on you in the moment.

··· QUIET CLASS: ROOM FOR YOUR MIND ···

Expound on Your Theme and Connect It to a Personal and a Universal Experience

Here's a not-so-secret secret: We don't always theme our classes. Sometimes we have distracted days, or frustrating days, or normal living-in-the-world days, and the theme we planned on "peace" doesn't feel like one we can offer with any degree of authenticity. When we feel this way, or when the world feels particularly full of strife, or the media is calling our attention to a tragedy of unimaginable scale, this is what we offer: silence. And more silence still.

Chants, Quotes, Mantras, Poems, or Songs That Connect

Wordless chanting: hum a single note, *m-m-m, m-m-m, m-m-m.*

If you typically have a playlist, opt out of music for this class.

Practices That Work with Your Theme

Yin yoga.

Multiple repetitions of a move, so you can say less as the teacher.

Familiar flows that require less cuing from you.

Forgoing music, or choosing mild instrumental music.

Distill Your Theme to a Short Sentence or Intention

Notice the silence as room for your mind.

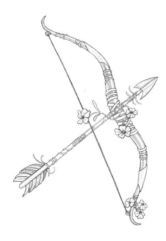

Phrases or Sentences to Employ in These Parts of Your Class

OPENING	DURING MOVEMENTS
Think of someone with whom you can have a peaceful silence while you eat, drive, or walk together: a dear friend or family member, perhaps. Now take the feelings that person evokes in you and turn them toward yourself in this practice. There's no need for self-talk as we go along. Let's revel in the comfortable quiet.	Notice the noise in the room—the music, your neighbors' breath. Can you let this soundtrack guide your practice even more, and let your mind go quiet?
DURING PAUSES	**CLOSING**
Sometimes when we settle in to the stillness in rest shapes like this, we find the mind ramps up. Can you exhale through your mouth—*ah-h-h*—to let those go, and invite in more quiet in your mind?	As you prepare to move back into the world of thinking and talking, consider that so many of us are inundated all day long with words, both written and spoken. Could you think ahead to some communication you need to deliver, and find the most kindly concise way to send it?

Takeaway Ideas

Ostensibly you are offering quiet because the world feels particularly harried or challenging that day. You might assume or intuit that your students feel the same and offer them something extra kind, like a small piece of chocolate on their mat as class ends.

Anything Else

The book *Smart Brevity: The Power of Saying More with Less,* by Jim VandeHei, Mike Allen, and Roy Schwartz (New York: Workman, 2022), is a pithy and clear guide to communicating more with less.

EFFORT AND EASE

Expound on Your Theme and Connect It to a Personal and a Universal Experience

Sthira sukham asanam: this is about the only instruction for asana that the sutras offer us. The pose—the seat—must have elements of effort, sthira, and elements of ease, sukha. Much of what we learn in the practice of yoga, physically, mentally, and spiritually, is where our efforts are best spent and where we might have room for more ease.

To everything there is a season. There's a time for putting in the work—for striving, for pushing, for making things happen. And there's a time to rest. As the mothers of daughters, we both know that there are some situations and conversations that require our input and effort, and others where offering ease and quiet— or self-censoring—is the better path. As Ecclesiastes says, there is "a time to keep silence, and a time to speak." The practice gives us tools to know which tack to take.

Chants, Quotes, Mantras, Poems, or Songs That Connect

Scripture: "To everything there is a season." —Ecclesiastes 3

Song: "Turn! Turn! Turn!" by The Byrds

Practices That Work with Your Theme

Repeating a shape in various relationships to gravity, some of which need more effort and others that allow for more ease.

Distill Your Theme to a Short Sentence or Intention

Meet the moment with the right energy.

Phrases or Sentences to Employ in These Parts of Your Class

OPENING	DURING MOVEMENTS
As you consider what brought you to your mat today and look ahead to the practice before us, think through whether you came to work or to rest. There's room for both throughout this class, and stating to yourself what you need is a chance to commit to your needs.	Now is the time for effort as we move. Even still, can you find the right amount of effort? It may be less, even far less, than you're currently using. If you can conserve your work here, you can push more somewhere else.
DURING PAUSES	**CLOSING**
As we rest here, the emphasis is clearly on ease. Notice, though, where you need to have a little control and apply effort. It might be directed toward keeping your attention in the here and now.	At the start of class, you thought through how much effort you'd need to expend, and how much ease you could allow. Now think ahead to the next few hours and strategize how you'll find the right balance so you can bring the right energy to meet each moment.

Takeaway Ideas

Since effort and ease are related but paradoxical ideas, you may offer your students a card that says "effort" on one side and "ease" on the other.

Anything Else

If you teach a variety of styles of yoga, this is an especially fun theme to employ across a spectrum of yoga classes.

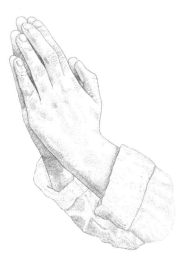

INTENTION FOLLOWS ACTION

Expound on Your Theme and Connect It to a Personal and a Universal Experience

We are *so* big on intention in yoga. We hear ourselves saying the word multiple times in every class, as we guide students to set and use an intention to shepherd them through the practice.

But sometimes we need to put the cart before the horse and just get going. Then the mood follows. Intention follows action.

This is how some workouts and writing sessions get done—and how, in our households, many meals get made. No, we don't feel like doing them. But we get started anyway. Sometimes we give ourselves permission to stop after ten minutes if things don't start to flow. They always do!

What a beautiful, freeing reminder for our students. However they showed up on their mats, they're in the right place. They can feel distracted, annoyed, still caught up in work, still ruminating on family life or child-rearing, and yet here they are, in yoga. If there is no clear intention, there doesn't have to be: The intention might arrive during class. The intention may show up in Savasana. The intention to come to the mat may be enough.

Chants, Quotes, Mantras, Poems, or Songs That Connect

Song: "Work Song" by Hozier

Song: "Sweet Life" by Essie Jain

Practices That Work with Your Theme

Cue the first portion of a familiar sequence (your usual warm-up, say, or Sun Salutations), and then let students fill in the next part with whatever feels right to them.

Distill Your Theme to a Short Sentence or Intention

Just get started.

Phrases or Sentences to Employ in These Parts of Your Class

OPENING	DURING MOVEMENTS
Maybe you already have a fully formed intention. Great! But today, let's also stay open to a secondary intention, something that can emerge when we get started.	What is this movement loosening up for you? Is an intention percolating?
DURING PAUSES	**CLOSING**
Now that we've let that shape or movement go, pause. Check in. Notice whether your intention has emerged to follow the action.	Can you think ahead to something that you aren't raring with excitement to undertake? And if so, can you commit, here and now, to getting started with it as soon as is feasible and giving it ten minutes of your time?

Takeaway Ideas

A piece of paper that could be used to write down first next steps toward that project that students considered in the closing of class.

Anything Else

Steve Magness, in *Do Hard Things: Why We Get Resilience Wrong and the Surprising Science of Real Toughness* (New York: HarperOne, 2022) and in much of his other work on peak performance, illustrates the importance of getting going and letting the mood follow.

A SPACE FOR MYSELF

Expound on Your Theme and Connect It to a Personal and a Universal Experience

One thing that consistently brings us to yoga or meditation is a desire to have a conversation with ourselves. This time to check in connects us to the important yogic practice of svadhyaya, or self-study. When we make time to tune out the world, we hear ourselves more.

One important aspect of this in the modern world is that a yoga class serves as a respite from technology. Teaching on this theme, we invite students to take off or silence smart watches and to recognize that they are happily free from the interruption of texts, emails, or other pressing tidbits of information. Instead, they get to be present in their bodies and with their breath, which feels somewhat novel in our era of continuous connection.

It can be helpful to acknowledge that students may either consciously or unconsciously have some nervousness about this internal turning—they may be unsure of what they'll find when they make the space to look within. You can remind them that their time on their mat and their practice both serve as an opportunity to greet their deepest selves, to check in with who they are today, to listen to their desires and meanderings without judgment and without restraint. This space they find for themselves makes them a stronger yoga practitioner, a better partner, friend, parent, student—whatever—and ultimately a better human.

Chants, Quotes, Mantras, Poems, or Songs That Connect

Song: "Slow Down" by Scott Orr

Song: "Ascent (Day 7)" by Ludovico Einaudi

Quote: "Loneliness is the poverty of self; solitude is the richness of self."
—May Sarton

Practices That Work with Your Theme

Poses that allow space for dropping into one's self, so obvious shapes like Child's Pose. But another sweet practice here is to try doing routine poses or sequences with your eyes closed. How does it change poses and movements like Downward-Facing Dog, a vinyasa sequence, or even just Cat and Cow when your attention is completely focused inward?

Humble Warrior and other forward folds may offer a physical sense of moving inward. In poses like Cobbler or Sphinx, having students drop their chin to their chest may offer that sense too.

Distill Your Theme to a Short Sentence or Intention

This is your space to drop into yourself.

Phrases or Sentences to Employ in These Parts of Your Class

OPENING	DURING MOVEMENTS
Your yoga practice is an opportunity to be in community with yourself. We'll begin with a seated breath practice. Let your mind roam freely, listening to what comes up. If you feel stuck in ruminant thoughts, return to your body and breath, letting your thoughts melt away. But if your thoughts flow freely, notice what they reveal to you.	Sometimes, when we move vigorously in a yoga practice, we don't get a chance to think. So here, as we balance and focus, check in. What's happening here in your mind? What do you find when you move inward here? Where have your thoughts naturally gone? Are you fully in this moment?
DURING PAUSES	CLOSING
We'll pause in silence now. Here, there is another opportunity to check in and notice what you are noticing. Here, there is a reminder that this is the work of doing nothing.	Your practice has been an opportunity to engage with your deepest self. As you move back into the world of connection and messages and interruptions, maybe give yourself a little more space and time before you check your email or before you read your text messages or before you reengage. Appreciate the important space of connection you have found with yourself through disconnection with technology.

Takeaway Ideas

Meditation instructions for a brief one- or two-minute breath check-in to revisit the quiet and connection found during the yoga practice.

Anything Else

Having space to yourself is a necessary kind of self-care. This theme reminds your students of that fact too.

7

ALIGNMENT LESSONS FOR ASANA AND LIFE

There are certain phrases yoga teachers love to say, not only because they apply to the physical poses, but also because they apply metaphysically as life lessons. Some of them are so mundane you probably haven't given them much thought as potential themes. In this chapter, we explore how these potentially trite cues that help us to align on the mat work as inspiration off the mat.

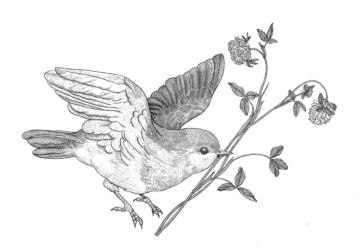

FOR MORE

More Themes to Explore

Soften your jaw.

Curl up the edges of your lips.

Trust your body.

Radiate from your core.

Lengthen through your spine.

Reading

Anatomy books can offer great sources of inspiration here. We love *Yoga Anatomy* by Leslie Kaminoff and Amy Matthews (Champaign, IL: Human Kinetics, 2022) and *Anatomy of Movement* by Blandine Calais-Germain (Seattle: Eastland Press, 1993).

LEAD WITH YOUR HEART

Expound on Your Theme and Connect It to a Personal and a Universal Experience

The common asana-class action cue, "Lead with your heart," is a reminder to keep a broad chest as you move from Mountain Pose into a forward fold. It's also a super reminder about the attitude you bring to every movement and every interaction across your day. Let's explore how this cue works both literally and metaphorically.

We know people often respond in kind to whatever energy you bring to any given interaction. If you show up loaded for bear—that is, ready to fight a giant adversary—you may wind up creating a contentious situation where you might not have otherwise. But when you meet each person with a sense of full-hearted openness, you're more often than not going to get that same energy back in return.

And this is true not only of your energy but also of your body language. When you're feeling closed off, it's common to cross your arms over your body. When you're feeling open, you instead spread them wide. When we practice leading with our hearts, both in movement and in relationships, we get better at using this open-hearted approach as our default mode.

Chants, Quotes, Mantras, Poems, or Songs That Connect

Poem: "Lead Me to the Song of My Heart" by Danna Faulds

Song: "Flying" by Garth Stevenson

Song: "I Forgive Myself & I Release" by Geminelle

Practices That Work with Your Theme

Backbends and heart openers. You could start class in a supported reclining backbend like Fish Pose on a bolster or blocks.

Distill Your Theme to a Short Sentence or Intention

Lead with your heart.

Phrases or Sentences to Employ in These Parts of Your Class

OPENING	DURING MOVEMENTS
As we settle into stillness in this supported backbend, can you think of a time you were feeling open and heart-centered? How does that feel in your body? How does your body respond to the memory? Let's try to grow this feeling in our practice today.	As you move through these rounds of Cat and Cow, notice the movement away from and toward an open-hearted position. How can you keep your awareness in this space?
DURING PAUSES	**CLOSING**
As we pause, try Puppy Pose instead of Child's Pose. Can you keep your heart open here?	Now as you prepare to move off the mat, can you think ahead to the next few hours? How can you lead with your heart as you spend time with your loved ones? Is there a situation in your near future where you might find it challenging to lead with your heart? How could you keep this openness and softness you cultivated today and carry it into this potentially challenging situation?

Takeaway Ideas

Anything heart-shaped. You could keep your eyes open after Valentine's Day to find little favors on deep discount!

Anything Else

This can be a sensitive theme for people feeling closed off or disconnected. Consider softening it from a directive, "Lead with your heart," to an investigation, "Do you want to lead with your heart?" or "How would it feel to lead with your heart?"

ROOT TO RISE

Expound on Your Theme and Connect It to a Personal and a Universal Experience

"Root to rise" is often given as a cue to press down to lift up: from forward fold to standing, up to Crow Pose, and so on. Newton's third law of motion tells us for every action there is an equal and opposite reaction. We must exert a downward force if we want to fly upward; we need to have something to press against.

The cue "Root to rise" also points to the importance of the infrastructure that underlies every action—from the growth of a tree, which depends on a deep root system, to the erection of a skyscraper, which needs a steady and stable base, to our feet, knees, and hips, which support us as we flow through asanas.

More metaphorically, we can consider how we need to have a base of stability undergirding our mobility and freedom. This ties right in to the concepts of sthira and sukha: The seat must be both steady and comfortable, both rooted and rising.

Chants, Quotes, Mantras, Poems, or Songs That Connect

Song: "No Roots" by Alice Merton

Song: "Opening" by East Forest

Chant: Rooted like a tree

Practices That Work with Your Theme

Anything that focuses on the feet and, when they are on the floor, the hands.

Distill Your Theme to a Short Sentence or Intention

Trust the ground.

Phrases or Sentences to Employ in These Parts of Your Class

OPENING	DURING MOVEMENTS
As we settle here, feel the solidness of the floor beneath your mat. Trust the ground to hold you and support your practice. Try letting go more into this support so you can free up energy to rise when we begin to move, faithful that the floor is always here for you.	Feel the support of the ground you enjoyed as we began. How is that giving you a base from which you can launch and reach upward?
DURING PAUSES	**CLOSING**
Send your roots down. Imagine each breath drawing in more nutrients as you settle and grow your potential.	As you prepare to move off the mat, reflect on what deep support you need to institute in order to reach upward toward your goals. What is the first next step toward implementing this support?

Takeaway Ideas

Offer your students cuttings from your garden or packets of seeds.

Anything Else

We love seeing more and more specialized yoga. Consider what a great theme this would be for a class just on yoga for feet!

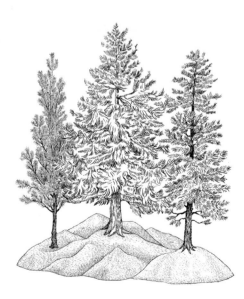

LESS IS MORE

Expound on Your Theme and Connect It to a Personal and a Universal Experience

Trying too hard is, by definition, counterproductive. We should aim instead to try just hard enough—to try right hard. We certainly feel this on the yoga mat. When you work too hard to get into a shape, your tensing up often makes the shape unsustainable. Thinking too hard about nailing a transition can prevent it from happening easily. And forcing a breath exercise to fit a particular rhythm that doesn't suit you can actually create agitation instead of relieving it.

We love to remind students that there is nothing sacred about the physical shapes we make in a yoga class—most of our modern asana practice was "invented" in the yoga revival of the late 1800s and early 1900s. And lithe men who were doing yoga for hours each day were by and large creating and performing the poses. That last tidbit is important because some of the alignment cues that linger on in our everyday classes no longer serve the bodies in the room: bodies that are often female, bodies that may sit for hours of a working day, bodies that would probably feel better in poses that are taught with less focus on rigid alignment. Less worry about doing it right—whether that's the asana or any other aspect of yoga—often means more revelation, freedom, and presence. Less is more, whether in rigidity of movement or thinking, or in effort.

Chants, Quotes, Mantras, Poems, or Songs That Connect

Poem: "Gentle" by Alfred K. LaMotte

Song: "Let It Be" by The Beatles

Song: "If You Love Somebody Set Them Free" by Sting

Practices That Work with Your Theme

Using props liberally! Set out one or two blankets for each student before they arrive.

Moving with soft joints: bent knees and elbows, for example.

Cue students into a pose, and cue them to back away from their full effort there.

Distill Your Theme to a Short Sentence or Intention

Hold the practice with an open hand.

You don't have to work so hard.

Phrases or Sentences to Employ in These Parts of Your Class

OPENING	DURING MOVEMENTS
Think of a time when you tried too hard. This could be anything from stripping a screw by applying too much pressure to driving someone away by clinging too much. Consider how today's practice can build on what you learned from that lesson.	What would it feel like to dial back your effort another 10 percent? Or even 20? How does that affect the experience? You can always add more work back.
DURING PAUSES	**CLOSING**
Settle into this rest and let it be. Notice if you're pushing even here, where there is no need.	Think ahead to a project you have coming up. Are there lessons from this practice that might help? Can you give yourself a mantra to help you remember that less is more?

Takeaway Ideas

Equip your students with a note card and pen and ask them to come up with a mantra that is similar to "less is more," but more personal to them. They get to create their own takeaway!

Anything Else

Encourage your students to learn more about yoga's history to disabuse them from any dogmatic, rigid approach to the practice or the poses. We love *Yoga Body: The Origins of Modern Posture Practice* (New York: Oxford University Press, 2010) by Mark Singleton.

MOVE INTO THE POSE PREPARED

Expound on Your Theme and Connect It to a Personal and a Universal Experience

As then-General Eisenhower said, when going into battle, "Plans are useless; planning is indispensable." Another military truism comes from a Prussian general, Helmuth von Moltke the Elder: "No plan of operations extends with any certainty beyond the first encounter with the main enemy forces." While it's critical to adapt to evolving situations in real time—and while the practice of yoga gives us the very tools of focus and presence that make this more doable—having thought ahead and planned a strategy is critically important.

This is true in asana practice, where we often carefully sequence the order of the poses so that the early ones prepare us for the latter. (For more about sequencing models, see Sage's 2024 book *The Art of Yoga Sequencing*.) Smart preparation lets us move into a pose prepared. In crucial, pivotal moments of the practice, we can see how our preparations with poses to strengthen, stretch, and warm us have readied us for where we've arrived. We sequence smartly not just to prepare for the poses that we know are coming, but to prepare for our time off the mat, where we can't predict what's going to happen at all. We can only do our best to prepare for the unexpected.

Chants, Quotes, Mantras, Poems, or Songs That Connect

Quote: "Everyone has a plan till they get hit." —Mike Tyson

Song: "Peaceful Groove" by Teen Daze

Practices That Work with Your Theme

Building to poses that require some preparation and assembly of constituent parts: an arm bind in a balance shape, for example.

Distill Your Theme to a Short Sentence or Intention

Are you ready?

Phrases or Sentences to Employ in These Parts of Your Class

OPENING	DURING MOVEMENTS
In our practice today, we're going to focus on the moment before movements: transitions. You'll notice that I cue a little more as we shift from one shape to another. This is to prepare you. Consider the cues and check in to see if you feel ready.	As we move into this shape, we're combining several of the actions we've already prepared. So as you move in, know that you already have succeeded, whether or not you get into the "full" pose.
DURING PAUSES	CLOSING
As you settle and rest, think back to that big shape we just took. You know you prepared physically for it. But take a moment to appreciate how your practice has prepared you in other ways to do that tricky thing and many others. Maybe you have learned to stay connected to your breath, or to go easy on yourself. What does your practice do to train you for life?	Remember again what the lessons your practice, today and over time, have conferred that work off the mat. As you prepare to step back into your life, recognize how your practice has helped you be more prepared.

Takeaway Ideas

The Girl Scout motto is "Be prepared." If you offered this theme at a time when those ubiquitous cookies were being offered for sale, you could share some with your students and offer them the motto as a connection to your theme.

Anything Else

There are a lot of philosophical places you could go with "preparation" as a theme. Consider that another way to look at this is that no matter how much we prepare, we can never be ready for all the shifts life offers us. It may be fun to offer this theme a few different ways.

······ YOUR TWO SIDES ARE DIFFERENT ······

Expound on Your Theme and Connect It to a Personal and a Universal Experience

As we move through life and asana, we are looking for balance, not symmetry. Your body is not symmetrical! Your heart is slightly to the left of center, and your lungs are shaped differently to accommodate this. You drive more (or exclusively) with your right foot, and you have a dominant hand. As anyone who has ever looked into a nonreversing mirror can attest, your face isn't symmetrical. You even have a dominant eye. So don't try to make your body symmetrical. Symmetry isn't our natural state or our natural way of existing, and it's not necessary for balance.

If you have two kids—or if you have a sibling—you know that even the very same pair of genes can combine differently instance to instance. You need to treat your children as you would treat your two sides: with equity, but not necessarily equality. In an asana practice, that means you may need to hold one side longer than the other until things feel right for you.

Chants, Quotes, Mantras, Poems, or Songs That Connect

Song: "Freedom" by Jon Batiste

Quote: "Don't confuse symmetry with balance." —Tom Robbins, *Even Cowgirls Get the Blues*

Practices That Work with Your Theme

Paying attention to both symmetrical and asymmetrical poses, perhaps by doing symmetrical shapes like Mountain or Chair in asymmetrical ways: lift one heel, lift only one arm.

Distill Your Theme to a Short Sentence or Intention

Meet each side where it is.

Phrases or Sentences to Employ in These Parts of Your Class

OPENING	DURING MOVEMENTS
As we get settled, notice whether your arrangement is symmetrical or asymmetrical. If you're sitting, which leg tucks in first? How would it feel to change this? If you're reclining, do the two sides of your body drop evenly into the floor, or can you notice differences?	Does this side feel the same as the first time we visited this shape? Do you have resistance to the difference? Can you notice how things are the same or different without judgment?
DURING PAUSES	**CLOSING**
As we rest here again, you may decide that this time or on this side you need more or less time in this pose. Stay longer if that's the case and join us in the practice when you feel that you've found what you needed here, remembering we aren't seeking symmetry but equity.	Can you conceive of differences in your body not as imbalances but as separate strengths? Or your body's specific sense of symmetry as a sort of superpower?

Takeaway Ideas

Equip your students with a note card and pen and have them draw an image that conjures up balance. Students may draw things like the yin-yang symbol or scales. Invite them to see their drawing as representative of the theme.

Anything Else

One fun movement practice to offer with this theme is to have your students walk up and down their mats with their eyes closed. Once they stop and take Mountain Pose, ask them to keep their eyes closed and invite them to notice how their body feels. Do they think their feet are pointed in the same direction? This little exercise can demonstrate a lot about our perception of balance and symmetry.

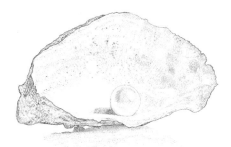

RELAX YOUR SHOULDERS

Expound on Your Theme and Connect It to a Personal and a Universal Experience

If you've ever seen Amy Cuddy's famous TED Talk on power posing,* you have learned how your body language influences your attitude. And while Cuddy's research has not been fully replicable, we know intuitively that there's truth to faking it until you make it. Cuddy calls it the "postural feedback effect."

Your body language also influences others' interpretation of your attitude. This is something we've already explored—that, as the teacher, you are likely telling yourself stories about what your students' facial expressions and body language mean, whether or not they are true stories.

We love Thich Nhat Hanh's notion of a half smile. The exercise, described in *The Miracle of Mindfulness,* involves consciously expressing a half smile on waking, in free moments, and when you're feeling irritated. Sage has found herself deploying this so often that, when she travels alone, she finds her face achy toward the end of the day because she has adopted a placid expression to keep herself relaxed and in control all day.

Chants, Quotes, Mantras, Poems, or Songs That Connect

Song: "Enchanted Forest" by Sol Rising

Chant: *Om mani padme hum:* The jewel is in the lotus flower of enlightenment.

Practices That Work with Your Theme

Experimenting with a variety of upper-body arrangements that key to body language: standing in Mountain Pose with your arms crossed versus open, for example.

Distill Your Theme to a Short Sentence or Intention

Let go and open up.

---

* Amy Cuddy, "Your Body Language May Shape Who You Are," TED, June 2012, www.ted.com/talks /amy_cuddy_your_body_language_may_shape_who_you_are.

Phrases or Sentences to Employ in These Parts of Your Class

OPENING	DURING MOVEMENTS
Let's start from a place of relaxing and opening. How could you arrange yourself right now to send a signal of openness and ease?	When your arms are lifted like this, your shoulders naturally lift too. See if you can relax there—or anywhere—without forcing them down. How can you be broad and open, and how does that affect your experience in the shape?
DURING PAUSES	CLOSING
This pause is a perfect time to relax your shoulders—and your forehead, and your jaw, and even your tongue, and anywhere else you're holding on. Let go.	What did you feel in the practice you'd like to carry out into the world? How can you express this with your physical body? Let's adopt these poses now, slowly open our eyes, and look around the room to see what others have cultivated.

Takeaway Ideas

A slip of paper with a reminder, "Drop your shoulders!"

Anything Else

You might include a neck stretching sequence or even a little shoulder and neck self-massage in service of your theme.

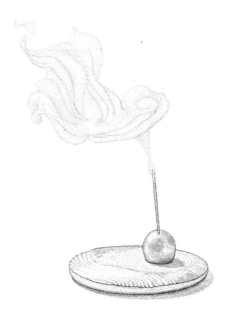

8

RISE TO JOY:
THEMES OF HAPPINESS

As the Greek playwright Aeschylus said, "Happiness is a choice that requires effort at times." By thinking about the conditions for happiness, and consciously orienting toward them, we can vastly improve our moods—and thus the moods of everyone around us.

In this chapter, we use themes from positive psychology that connect to yoga. Since the point and purpose of yoga is to connect more deeply with your truest self and be more liberated, it's not a stretch to say that yoga's goal is to increase your joy. Life is fleeting; we are here to help others and to spread love. But surely, we are also here to experience delight!

FOR MORE

More Themes to Explore

There are so many words for happiness, and they all connote slightly different things. How would you theme differently on sukha, jubilation, cheer, *ananda*, contentment, delight, glee, enjoyment, or merriment? Rather than think of happiness as one emotion, consider that it is a facet of many emotions. How do we tap into these different experiences of joy? Could you create a month of themes that asked students to meditate on these experiences of bliss?

Reading

Ali Abdaal, *Feel-Good Productivity: How to Do More of What Matters to You* (Stevens Point, WI: Cornerstone, 2023).

Kristin Neff, *Self-Compassion: The Proven Power of Being Kind to Yourself* (New York: William Morrow, 2011).

Thich Nhat Hanh, *The Miracle of Mindfulness* (Boston: Beacon, 1975).

Dalai Lama, *The Art of Happiness: A Handbook for Living* (New York: Penguin, 2009).

PRACTICE GRATITUDE

Expound on Your Theme and Connect It to a Personal and a Universal Experience

This is no longer news to anyone: Positive psychology teaches us the importance of a gratitude practice for a happy life. But like getting at least eight hours of sleep and eating enough vegetables, just because we know something is good for us doesn't mean we do it. Students will be familiar with the idea of a gratitude practice, but that doesn't mean they have one or they have even formally engaged in gratitude *as* a practice. This theme is valuable for that reason: It can serve as an opportunity to show students how easy and helpful it is to take a few moments to be grateful.

Approach this by either asking students to take time at the start of class to write about what they feel grateful for this day or guide them through this as they settle into class.

Chants, Quotes, Mantras, Poems, or Songs That Connect

Quote: "Yes, thanks." —Thich Nhat Hanh, *The Miracle of Mindfulness*

Poem: "Happiness" by Stephen Dunn

Song: "Thank You" by Beautiful Chorus

Practices That Work with Your Theme

Poses that ask you to bow forward, like Humbled Warrior or Wide-Legged Standing Forward Fold, offer an opportunity to express physical thankfulness.

Distill Your Theme to a Short Sentence or Intention

Thank you so much.

Phrases or Sentences to Employ in These Parts of Your Class

OPENING	DURING MOVEMENTS
As you settle in, take stock of your raw materials. What are you working with today? Does your attention go straight to spots of tightness, tension, or tiredness? It's good to notice them so you can make smart choices around them when we come into movement. But please focus now on the good. What already feels decent? If you get really granular—like right hand, ring finger, second knuckle—you'll quickly have a long inventory of things to feel grateful for.	Move through this next round of poses with a grateful heart. You get to be here! You get to do this! You are healthy and strong enough to be here on your mat, moving and breathing and feeling connected.
DURING PAUSES	**CLOSING**
You might like to offer a sigh of gratitude, giving thanks for your body and your breath.	Think ahead to some project that feels complex. Can you take the time here to feel grateful for all the skills you have developed that will help you tackle this project? Some of these skills might come right from your practice. Thank yourself for taking this time to hone your skills.

Takeaway Ideas

You could offer your students any small token that expresses your gratitude for them. Or, if you have students write about what they are grateful for as part of the class, they will leave with their gratitude list. You could also follow up with an email that explains how to create a daily gratitude list practice.

Anything Else

While this is a theme you can offer to students to think about, it may be a more meaningful theme if you set aside some materials for writing out a gratitude list. You could start practice this way, inviting students to gather a piece of paper and pen on their way into class.

Before students begin, or as they are starting to write, share what's on your list, offering a model for them. Offer a mix of serious and nonserious, material and immaterial so that they are guided to what's most meaningful to them.

HAPPINESS AND THE HARDER EMOTIONS

Expound on Your Theme and Connect It to a Personal and a Universal Experience

It's valuable to theme on the idea that harder emotions, like sadness and anger, are the other sides of the coin when it comes to happiness. As the poet John Keats tells us, "in the very temple of Delight / veil'd Melancholy has her sovran shrine." Since theming on happiness to any degree will mean that your students reflect on their own state of happiness, reminding them that the path toward happiness winds through the forest of grief, anger, or even resentment can offer them an out if they aren't feeling abundant joy the day you happen to share this theme.

Another way to consider this is that all emotions are part of life. We can't have happiness without having all the attendant emotions of existence. In Coleman Barks's translation of Islamic mystic Jalaluddin Rumi's poem "The Guest House," the poet tells us to imagine all of our emotions are treasured guests to be invited in as honored guests into our home: "The dark thought, the shame, the malice, / meet them at the door laughing, / and invite them in."

It may seem contradictory to theme a practice on emotions that are the opposite of joy, but that's sort of the point: When we remember that happiness is not the zenith of some tall mountain, but rather the vistas along a path that has many lovely peaks and some valleys, we are better equipped to traverse the valleys.

Chants, Quotes, Mantras, Poems, or Songs That Connect

Poem: "Ode on Melancholy" by John Keats

Poem: "The Guest House" by Jalaluddin Rumi, translated by Coleman Barks

Practices That Work with Your Theme

In seated or supine poses, invite students to stack their hands over their hearts in a gesture of connection to themselves and self-compassion for whatever their feelings might be.

Play with movements that explore heart-opening and closing: spinning in and out of Thread-the-Needle, or Downward-Facing Dog to Wild Thing.

Distill Your Theme to a Short Sentence or Intention

Wherever your emotions are today, happiness is somewhere on your path.

Phrases or Sentences to Employ in These Parts of Your Class

OPENING	DURING MOVEMENTS
Wouldn't it be nice to live in a state of happiness? I hope you are feeling happy today, but if you showed up on your mat processing a harder emotion, I want to invite you to be fully present with how you're feeling today, knowing that this is just part of the path.	Notice the flow state you're in here while moving. Where are your emotions now?
DURING PAUSES	**CLOSING**
Pauses give you a chance to check in, to listen to your body's wisdom. Is there a message here that connects to how you showed up today?	As you allow your body to drift into Savasana, invite in any emotional guests that come to visit.

Takeaway Ideas

We love the symbolism of gemstones. Small pieces of pink quartz or pyrite can remind students of their abiding happiness, which they will find again. You can also offer copies of a poem like Rumi's "The Guest House," or Keats's "Ode on Melancholy."

Anything Else

Sometimes students have emotional responses to messages. The art of holding space means that you meet students wherever they are, make eye contact, and don't rush them through whatever response they are having.

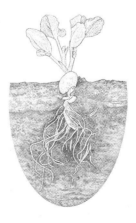

PROTECT YOUR BOUNDARIES

Expound on Your Theme and Connect It to a Personal and a Universal Experience

It's easy to have boundaries when you're alone. It's harder when you're faced with a person or a circumstance that invites you to let those boundaries slide. Your practice can be a laboratory in which you experiment with establishing and then holding your boundaries. It can build your resistance and clarity in tempting situations.

For example, if there's a pose or category of poses that you know aggravates an injury, you could practice committing to not doing them, even if everyone else in the room does. Sometimes telling your teacher, or your neighbor, that you are opting out makes it easier to hold your boundaries and not get swept up.

Chants, Quotes, Mantras, Poems, or Songs That Connect

Aphorism: What you allow will continue.

Song: "Wise Up" by Aimee Mann

Song: "happiness" by Taylor Swift

Practices That Work with Your Theme

Anything taught in stages, where there's always a next-level variation to mention. Invite students not to proceed through all the steps, and instead to pause at their own best spot.

Have students practice *abhaya mudra,* which sort of looks like holding a hand up to gesture "stop." It's often seen in depictions of Hindu deities or the Buddha and it's used to symbolize protection.

Distill Your Theme to a Short Sentence or Intention

Not today.

Phrases or Sentences to Employ in These Parts of Your Class

OPENING	DURING MOVEMENTS
Think through a situation in your life where you are frequently tempted—or imposed upon—to cede your boundaries. Maybe you can't walk past a coffee shop without buying a latte; maybe you can't say no to a particular coworker who imposes on your kindness by piling tasks onto your plate. Imagine saying, "Not today," and holding firm. Let's see if we can carry this energy through the practice.	Check in with your intention. Are you staying within your boundaries?
DURING PAUSES	**CLOSING**
Take the time here to recharge your battery, so you can hold your boundaries firmly.	When you say no to people or things that impose on your time and goodwill, you're saying yes to something else. Take a moment here to consider what you want to say yes to. Now think though what might need a *no* so that can happen.

Takeaway Ideas

Since *yes* and *no* are key phrases for this theme, consider offering students a note card that says this—one word on each side.

Anything Else

Nedra Glover Tawwab's *Set Boundaries, Find Peace: A Guide to Reclaiming Yourself* (New York: TarcherPerigee, 2021) is a great book on holding firm boundaries for your mental health.

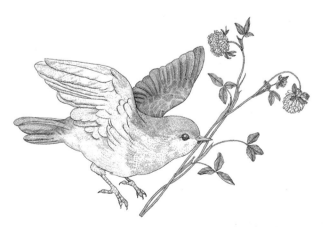

···· HAPPINESS IS A PRACTICE (MUDITA) ····

Expound on Your Theme and Connect It to a Personal and a Universal Experience

We sometimes imagine the path to happiness as a checklist: work out, eat healthy, go to therapy, read for forty-five minutes a day, do a morning ice plunge—or whatever is on your checklist. But what if the only thing on the checklist was "Be happy"? What if, instead of imagining we could bargain our way to happiness through endless action, we saw happiness itself as the practice? This radical notion is at the heart of *mudita*.

Author Kurt Vonnegut frequently told a story about his Uncle Alex, who made it a point to notice when he was happy. "His principal complaint about other human beings," Vonnegut reports, "was that they so seldom noticed it when they were happy. So when we were drinking lemonade under an apple tree in the summer, say, and talking lazily about this and that, almost buzzing like honeybees, Uncle Alex would suddenly interrupt the agreeable blather to exclaim, 'If this isn't nice, I don't know what is.'" Vonnegut told his audience, "I urge you to please notice when you are happy, and exclaim or murmur or think at some point, 'If this isn't nice, I don't know what is.'"*

Often happiness is more closely available to us than we realize. This isn't to suggest we can will ourselves to be happy in bad circumstances or that we should pretend or grin and bear it. But sometimes we get so caught up in doing, being, planning, growing, making, and fixing that we forget to simply notice the simple, easy joy that is already present.

Chants, Quotes, Mantras, Poems, or Songs That Connect

Quote: "If this isn't nice, I don't know what is." —Kurt Vonnegut

Song: "Shri" by DJ Drez

Song: "Joy (Unspeakable)" by Voices of Fire

---

* Kurt Vonnegut, *A Man Without a Country* (New York: Random House, 2005).

Practices That Work with Your Theme

Add an extra breath, or more, in each shape that gives you time to appreciate the good.

Teach a sequence and then have students move through it on their own, with limited cuing from you, following their own bliss.

Distill Your Theme to a Short Sentence or Intention

The first practice of happiness is noticing your own joy.

Phrases or Sentences to Employ in These Parts of Your Class

OPENING	DURING MOVEMENTS
You get a chance in our practice to notice what you notice. Let your intention be to notice moments of joy.	As we move through this sequence again, where do you feel light and free? Where do you feel joyous and at one with your breath and body?
DURING PAUSES	**CLOSING**
If this moment isn't nice, adjust your body until it is. Marinate in the satisfaction and comfort of this pause.	Before you begin to move your body out of this relaxation pose, take a moment to think to yourself, "If this isn't nice, I don't know what is."

Takeaway Ideas

Make a point of offering each of your students a smile (or maybe even a hug!) as they pack up and make their way out the door.

Anything Else

Another form of happiness is *maitri:* happiness specifically in relation to others' joy—the opposite of schadenfreude. Share this idea with your students too, and invite them to connect with their yoga neighbor by sharing something they feel grateful for with another student in the class.

FEED HEALTHY DISTRACTIONS

Expound on Your Theme and Connect It to a Personal and a Universal Experience

Both of us were very busy with other projects while drafting this book. This meant we could use our procrastination on the manuscript to direct focus to our other projects—leading yoga teacher training for Alexandra, developing the Two Weeks to Transformation retreat for Sage. In fact, we know productive procrastination to be such a powerful technique that we intentionally block out periods of focused work on multiple fronts. (Our houses have never been so clean, for example.)

In your life, is there something you turn to as a procrastination tool that winds up being a healthy distraction? For example, do you clean your house or meal prep in times of stress? That's a net win! It's amazing how compelling bathroom drawer-organizing can suddenly feel when the alternative is sitting down with a big project. These are the types of healthy distractions we love: reading a good book, even though there is laundry to do; working out, even if there's a wealth of emails in the inbox; taking time to be present with your family, even when the to-do list seems endless.

And neuroscience shows that often this kind of diversion is just what your mind needs to come up with creative solutions to your problems.[*] It's the revelation that comes to you in the shower, or the perfect phrase you construct while out on your walk. Your yoga practice can be exactly the time and place where your brain is forging deeper connections—and all while you relax, move, and breathe.

Chants, Quotes, Mantras, Poems, or Songs That Connect

Song: "Kothbiro" by Ayub Ogada

Song: "Sunrise" by Norah Jones

Practices That Work with Your Theme

Long rest periods.

Fun, creative arm variations that distract from long holds in lunges or Chair.

---

[*] Richard Sima, "Why Do We Get Our Best Ideas in the Shower?" *Washington Post,* January 12, 2023, www.washingtonpost.com/wellness/2023/01/12/shower-thoughts-creativity-brain.

Distill Your Theme to a Short Sentence or Intention

Lean in to this moment.

Phrases or Sentences to Employ in These Parts of Your Class

OPENING	DURING MOVEMENTS
Maybe today's practice is filling this role of a healthy distraction for you. Great! Take a moment to turn away from that project you're avoiding and to turn toward this pleasant procrastination practice. Know that often it's when you turn away from something that you're chewing on that breakthroughs occur.	Where do you feel the most effort in this shape? Where do you feel the least? Can you redirect your attention to the areas that aren't working hard? Notice how that affects your experience in this pose.
DURING PAUSES	**CLOSING**
Settle in, turning away from the work you just did. There's no need to think about the next round, the next pose, the next project.	Think ahead to a project you'll be working on soon. Can you strategize some healthy distractions you can turn to when you feel like you're hitting dead ends? And can you link your plans to a word or phrase you can use as a mantra?

Takeaway Ideas

Invite students to compile a "healthy distractions" playlist by sending you their favorite distraction songs. Compile this and share it via email or newsletter with your students.

Anything Else

If your students are unfamiliar with the idea of "productive procrastination" (accomplishment and avoidance all packaged up nicely), share this concept with them. They may recognize it in themselves.

LOVING KINDNESS (METTA)

Expound on Your Theme and Connect It to a Personal and a Universal Experience

To get better at anything, from cooking to playing an instrument to speaking a language, you have to practice. We might like to run a marathon, for example, but just saying we want to isn't enough. We also have to form a plan and enact that plan! To get better at being loving, kind, and compassionate, you also have to practice. Just like you'd follow a training plan to get ready for a race of any distance, sending loving kindness, known as *metta*, is a workout to build your capacity to love.

We all need to practice loving kindness. And, like running, it gets easier with repetition. Sending loving kindness is a beautiful layer to add into classes of every intensity level, from restorative to yoga malas (108 consecutive Sun Salutations).

To practice metta, visualize several people in various categories and send them love and well wishes, using this mantra: *May you be happy. May you be healthy. May you be whole.*

As a seated meditation, we usually practice sending loving kindness to people in four categories: ourselves, loved ones, neutral figures, and problematic people. In yoga, we euphemistically call those in the last category "precious jewels," as they offer the greatest opportunity to grow our loving kindness. When we practice metta in motion, we can be working with one individual all class or cycle through any or all of the four categories.

Chants, Quotes, Mantras, Poems, or Songs That Connect

Song: "All You Need Is Love" by the Beatles

Song: "My Love Mine All Mine" by Mitski

Song: "Real Love Baby" by Father John Misty

Chant: *Lokah samastah sukhino bhavantu:* May all beings everywhere be happy and free.

Practices That Work with Your Theme

Supported backbends and any open-hearted pose.

Child's Pose, for self-love.

Standing facing different directions in the room, imagining sending metta in these various directions.

As you chant *Lokah samastah sukhino bhavantu*, explain the meaning and invite students to tap into the love they've generated.

Distill Your Theme to a Short Sentence or Intention

May you be happy. May you be healthy. May you be whole.

Phrases or Sentences to Employ in These Parts of Your Class

OPENING	DURING MOVEMENTS
Being loving and kind takes *work!* Just as you can't sit on the sofa and get faster at running, you can't expect to be a more loving and kind person without practicing.	Keep your heart open.
	Don't close off to love.
Think of a time in your life when you felt really loving. Maybe think of the honeymoon period of a new romance, or the way it feels to adopt a pet. Where does that feeling show up in your body? Let's start sending loving kindness to the recipient of this love—someone you have already had practice adoring. Visualize them clearly. Now send them metta: May you be happy. May you be healthy. May you be whole.	Imagine someone you love doing this pose in a mirror image in your line of sight. Send them metta: May you be happy. May you be healthy. May you be whole.

DURING PAUSES	CLOSING
Notice what's shifting as you stay open, kind, and loving. Is there a change in your response depending on whom you're sending metta toward?	Think of a "precious jewel," someone who can feel tough to love. There's no need to choose your mortal enemy; just draw up the image of someone you find challenging. Take a deep breath and relax any tension that has crept in. Now send this person metta, just like you've been doing all class. Notice how this sits in your body.
	The next time you find yourself feeling less than kind, less than loving, engage in a round or two of metta. You can start with people who are easy to love and work up from there. You can do this any time, day or night, and it's a nice practice to remember if you are lying awake or have some unexpected downtime in your day.

Takeaway Ideas

A card with the metta mantra.

Written instructions or an audio or video of recorded full four-round metta meditation.

Anything Else

This makes an especially great theme to revisit over the course of a month or so, so students can feel how it gets easier with practice. This is an obvious theme to use around Valentine's Day.

The concept of loving kindness reminds us, as Southerners, of the popular phrase "Bless your heart!" While it's often used snidely as an oblique put-down, it's also used genuinely as an expression of loving kindness, in recognition of someone's finer qualities or good intentions. The Dharma Punx notably distill the metta mantra to "I love you. Keep going." Feel free to offer that to your students if it feels more natural.

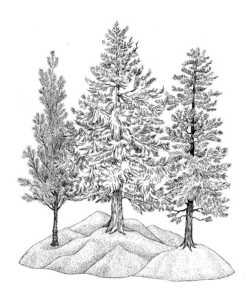

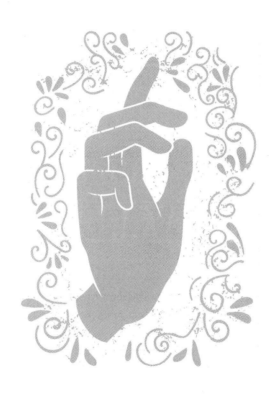

9

THEMES FROM HINDU MYTHOLOGY AND STORIES

Hindu stories are a part of yoga. So many pose names grow out of this beautiful faith tradition and are worthy of exploration. Consider how enriching it would be for your students to understand why Natarajasana is Dancer Pose! Many of the holidays celebrated in Indian culture, like Holi, Diwali, and Maha Shivaratri, have roots in Hindu deity myths and stories. Learning about these holidays and sharing the stories they arise from is a way to respectfully pay homage to the roots of yoga.

FOR MORE

More Themes to Explore

Learn the story of Nataraj, an avatar of Shiva, and the sages Vishvamitra and Vashista, and share those stories alongside the poses Natarajasana, Vishvamitrasana, and Vashistasana.

Learn about Hindu creation stories and develop themes that allow you to share what you've learned.

There are a vast number of stories about avatars of Shakti or other female deities like Parvati, Durga, Lakshmi, and Saraswati that the women in your classes may especially love to learn about.

Reading

Raj Balkaran, *The Stories Behind the Poses: The Indian Mythology That Inspired 50 Yoga Postures* (Brighton, UK: Leaping Hare, 2022)

Alanna Kaivalya and Arjuna van der Kooij, *Myths of the Asanas: The Ancient Origins of Yoga* (San Rafael, CA: Mandala, 2010)

Sanjay Patel, *The Little Book of Hindu Deities: From the Goddess of Wealth to the Sacred Cow* (London: Plume, 2006)

······ MATSYA: HUMANITY'S LIFEGUARD ······

Expound on Your Theme and Connect It to a Personal and a Universal Experience

Like many faith traditions, there is a parable of a great flood in Hinduism. In one story, Vishnu takes the form of Matsya and proceeds to save great sacred texts, the Vedas, from being lost. Even more importantly, Matsya also saves King Manu from the great flood, allowing him to go on to grow human existence. In both instances, Matsya models effortless giving on behalf of humanity.

We are often called to yoga because it makes *us* feel better. Consider that you first came to the practice not because it did anything for your neighbor, but because you slept better, felt better, and discovered more ease in your thoughts and movements. Ultimately, though, your yoga practice serves others too. When you step off the mat, you are a kinder, more present, more self-aware version of yourself, and thus better equipped to love your neighbor, help a stranger, and open your heart to the community around you. Yoga is not the answer to the world's problems, but peaceful practices of all kinds ultimately plant the seeds from which peace grows.

In this way, your time on the mat can be the start of mindful service to others. The model of Matsya allows us to ask ourselves, in what way am I serving humanity? Is there room for me to give more in large or small ways?

Chants, Quotes, Mantras, Poems, or Songs That Connect

Song: "Human Qualities" by Explosions in the Sky

Chant: *So hum:* oneness

Quote: "The greatness of a community is most accurately measured by the compassionate actions of its members." —Coretta Scott King

Practices That Work with Your Theme

Start or end the practice in supported Fish Pose. Explore any versions of Matsyasana and Matsyendrasana.

Distill Your Theme to a Short Sentence or Intention

How does your yoga serve your community?

Phrases or Sentences to Employ in These Parts of Your Class

OPENING	DURING MOVEMENTS
Your practice gives you a chance to give to yourself. Take a moment to reflect on who else reaps the benefit of your dedication to this intentional time.	The focus required to shift from this pose to the next one may feel like an activity tied just to this moment, but can you see how this practice of focus and presence now may show up later in service to others?
DURING PAUSES	**CLOSING**
Take the deepest breath here—maybe the deepest breath you've taken yet in our practice. While this experience is yours alone, you are breathing in a space with others.	Your path off the mat takes you back into a community of others: people you can help and connect with.

Takeaway Ideas

Consider pairing this practice with a business-savvy but theme-appropriate practice: Offer your students a card or pass for a free class if they bring a friend.

Anything Else

Since yoga as a community practice is a foundation for this theme, it may be sweet to end practice by asking students to take a moment of quiet gratitude for the people or circumstances that made their class attendance today possible.

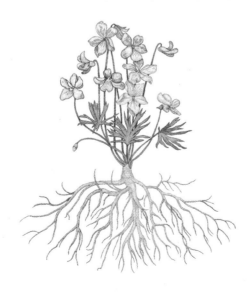

AGNI: PURIFICATION THROUGH DESTRUCTION

Expound on Your Theme and Connect It to a Personal and a Universal Experience

Agni, or fire, is an ancient god from Hindu stories that plays many roles: Agni is the fire of digestion, the fire in all humans, and the fire of transformation. Agni's many roles are familiar ones. We know fire can destroy and it can nurture. It can transmute.

Fire is necessary to remove the underbrush in the forest. This underbrush can choke out trees, ultimately destroying the forest. Periodic wildfires that purge the brush are critical to the overall health of the ecosystem. Just like a beautiful forest, our lives sometimes need purging, deep cleaning, a ritual, routine, and controlled burning.

Chants, Quotes, Mantras, Poems, or Songs That Connect

Song: "I Need a Forest Fire" by James Blake

Quote: "Each of us is born with a box of matches inside us but we can't strike them all by ourselves." —Laura Esquivel, *Like Water for Chocolate*

Practices That Work with Your Theme

Kapalabhati, or other breath exercises that build heat.

Kriya-type movements, like coming in and out of squat or in and out of a twist.

Distill Your Theme to a Short Sentence or Intention

Let it burn.

Phrases or Sentences to Employ in These Parts of Your Class

OPENING	DURING MOVEMENTS
With a practice themed around fire, there'll be some options tonight to stoke the flame high. Before we begin, please take the time to check in and make your own boundaries clear to yourself. Given the day and week you've had, the state of your body and mind, and anything you've got coming up soon, you may be burning with zeal. Or you may want to pull back away from the fire. Imagine just where you'd want to set up if we were sitting around a campfire. Make this your intention for practice.	There's heat building here! Can you let this heat temper you, purify you, change you into your essence? Or, if you're burning up, can you pull back a little so you're finding just the right temperature?
DURING PAUSES	**CLOSING**
Rest. Let the fire burn down some. You can always stoke it again.	Think of an ember from this practice that you'd like to carry forward, something you can stoke into a flame in the future.

Takeaway Ideas

Consider other images that connect to this theme; fire, salamanders, or phoenixes come to mind. Offer your students a stamped card with a flame image or something similar.

Anything Else

Agni is often depicted with two heads: one depicts immortality and preservation, the other mortality, death, and destruction. If you can bring in an image or *murti* of this deity, do!

HANUMAN: LOYALTY AS A VIRTUE

Expound on Your Theme and Connect It to a Personal and a Universal Experience

Hanuman is the monkey god whose absolute dedication to the king, Rama, was revered. He's come to symbolize great loyalty, and the pose associated with him, Hanumanasana, or Full Split Pose, is certainly one that requires deep commitment.

What does loyalty mean to you? Who are you loyal to? Yourself? In the context of a yoga practice, consider what loyalty to yourself might mean. For instance, it may look like prioritizing your body's needs rather than doing the practice exactly as it's offered. It may look like practicing a pose you are excited about routinely until you can do it with ease. Loyalty may look like showing up for your practice, whether that's physical asana, meditation, or some other variety of yoga practice, even when you're exhausted or disinterested.

Chants, Quotes, Mantras, Poems, or Songs That Connect

Song: "Jai Hanuman" by Craig Kohland and Shaman's Dream

Song: "Strength Courage & Wisdom" by India.Arie

Practices That Work with Your Theme

There is so much to play with in Hanumanasana, or Full Split Pose. You might explore variations of Ardha Hanumanasana, Half Split, or even teach a series of classes on dedication and loyalty where you build up to a Full Split practice.

Distill Your Theme to a Short Sentence or Intention

Be loyal to yourself.

Phrases or Sentences to Employ in These Parts of Your Class

OPENING	DURING MOVEMENTS
Employ loyalty as we move today. Be loyal to your body. Be loyal to your energetic needs.	Does your body want to do this next pose? Does your mind?
DURING PAUSES	**CLOSING**
Do you want to stay here longer? What do you need here?	You've listened to yourself and acted in accordance with your own needs; that's an act of brave self-loyalty that you can take off the mat. What does that look like outside this room?

Takeaway Ideas

Since Hanuman is the monkey god, offer your students any little monkey talisman you can think of.

Anything Else

The story of Hanuman comes from the Ramayana, an ancient Indian epic poem centered on Prince Rama (who is also a deity) and his wife Sita. Hanuman is a central character of the tale. There are many translations and variations on this story. One extremely approachable version we love is Sanjay Patel's beautifully illustrated modern retelling, *Ramayana: Divine Loophole* (San Francisco: Chronicle, 2010). And the animated movie *Sita Sings the Blues* is another appealing version of the story.

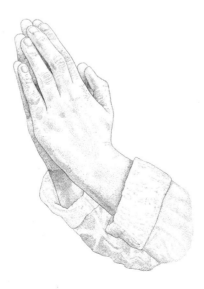

KALI: THE CYCLE OF LIFE

Expound on Your Theme and Connect It to a Personal and a Universal Experience

The cycle of creation-preservation-destruction defines existence. It's the larger cycle of our lives, and it also plays out in microcosmic ways, like in the reproductive cycle women experience monthly. But whether you identify as a woman or not, the familiar cycle of creation to destruction is omnipresent. From each relationship that ends sprouts the seed for the next one to begin. Each job interview with no forthcoming offer opens the door to the next perfect career fit. Each moment of despair or hurt enlarges your capacity for joy and love later. These cycles are the cycles of everyone's life experience.

In the space of a yoga practice, we can recognize that everything has a beginning, middle, and end: poses, breaths, states of being. Draw your students' attention to this through the practice.

Chants, Quotes, Mantras, Poems, or Songs That Connect

Song: "Soulful" by L'indécis

Song: "Love More" by Sharon Van Etten

Quote: "Birth is painful and delightful. Death is painful and delightful. Everything that ends is also the beginning of something else. Pain is not a punishment; pleasure is not a reward." —Pema Chödrön, *When Things Fall Apart: Heart Advice for Difficult Times*

Quote: "Grapes. Unripe . . . ripened . . . then raisins. Constant transitions, not the 'not' but the 'not yet.'" —Marcus Aurelius, *Meditations,* translated by Gregory Hays

Practices That Work with Your Theme

Flowing movements repeated in cycles, with discernible beginnings, middles, and ends.

Encourage your students to notice each part of their breath cycle and to explore shortening or lengthening their inhalations and exhalations.

Distill Your Theme to a Short Sentence or Intention

Beginning, middle, and end.

Phrases or Sentences to Employ in These Parts of Your Class

OPENING	DURING MOVEMENTS
This is the opening, the start to our practice. *Atha yoga anushasanam.* What does it feel like to begin? Hopeful? Relieving? What emotions reside in the start of things?	This movement has a beginning, a middle, and an end. Can you feel the moment when one yields to the next? Are you drawn more toward the initiation, the sustaining, or the finish of the movement? Can you smooth them out so they are balanced?
DURING PAUSES	**CLOSING**
This rest might feel like the end of the work. But notice that it's a chance for you to gather up your energy to begin again, and it's a shape in its own right. All the elements of the cycle are here.	Class is coming to an end, which means something new is about to begin. As you think ahead to this next thing, can you find some lesson from this practice that will help you be more present as the cycle plays out?

Takeaway Ideas

Simple hand-drawn talismans can be very powerful. Offer your students little line drawings of images that represent this cycle, such as three arrows moving in a circle.

Anything Else

This idea of birth/creation–preservation/sustenance–death/destruction plays out in deities Brahma-Vishnu-Shiva, the Trimurti.

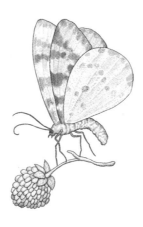

PARVATI: DEVOTION AND COMMITMENT

Expound on Your Theme and Connect It to a Personal and a Universal Experience

Parvati is an incarnation of Shakti and is most known as Shiva's consort. In Hindu myths and stories, our favorite depictions of her are when she seems like a typical, loving, but distracted spouse—she half-listens to Shiva, she notices when he espouses things she already knows, she loves him despite his flaws. Her love isn't aspirational; it's typical. It's a reminder that the love you feel for your partner, your family, or your friends is what it means to be human. Devotion and commitment are not lofty notions only for the gods; rather they are the requisites for fulfilling and loving relationships with the people in your life. When you love from a place of authenticity, devotion and commitment come with ease.

Your yoga practice is a solo pursuit, where you can practice devotion and commitment in relation to yourself. What does it mean to have a practice that is full of self-devotion? That is unequivocally committed to your needs?

Chants, Quotes, Mantras, Poems, or Songs That Connect

Poem: "I Loved You Before I Was Born" by Li-Young Lee

Song: "Devotion" by Indigo Girls

Song: "Fallin'" by Alicia Keys

Practices That Work with Your Theme

A practice supported by props. Treat yourself as a beloved partner and offer yourself the support of the props!

Distill Your Theme to a Short Sentence or Intention

Let your practice arise from self-love.

Phrases or Sentences to Employ in These Parts of Your Class

OPENING	DURING MOVEMENTS
Take a moment to greet yourself. By showing up, you've demonstrated your devotion to your practice and yourself.	How can you be a consort to yourself? How can you provide yourself some cheerleading support? Or do you need to gently remind yourself you could be doing more here?
DURING PAUSES	**CLOSING**
Can your breath be your helpmate here, standing close at hand to offer exactly what you need?	As you prepare to move off the mat, consider the marriage of your body, mind, and breath. Can you recommit to this partnership? Yoga is this union of your self and your Self.

Takeaway Ideas

Offer each of your students a length of ribbon that would fit around their wrist or ankle, with the suggestion that they tie it on and wear it as a reminder of their devotion to themselves.

Anything Else

For this theme we extrapolated on the devotion that Parvati shows in partnership and applied it to devotion to self. But talking about Parvati's devotion to Shiva may be a beautiful theme for a partner yoga or couple-specific class.

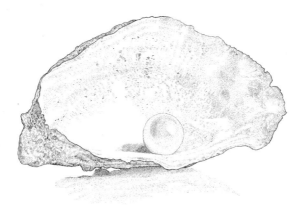

DURGA: FEARLESSNESS

Expound on Your Theme and Connect It to a Personal and a Universal Experience

Feel afraid? Do it anyway. Durga is a fierce warrior, and she's often depicted riding around on tigers and other predators. She's not afraid, though, because she doesn't need to be: She knows that she is powerful over her enemies, and her true power radiates from within. That's the lesson of Durga: When we want something badly enough, we act despite our fears.

Alexandra's elementary-aged daughter recently got her ears pierced. While she very much wanted to wear earrings, she agonized over whether the piercings would be painful. She was afraid, but squeezed her eyes shut and quietly announced, after the first ear was pierced, "It's not that bad," and then she laughed and laughed, mostly out of relief.

This example of Durga's fierceness is a reminder that we have to face our fears; we can feel nervous and choose to move forward in spite of that. After all, if we waited until we had absolutely no fear, we wouldn't do much at all.

Chants, Quotes, Mantras, Poems, or Songs That Connect

Aphorism: Speak the truth, even if your voice shakes.

Song: "Brave" by Sara Bareilles

Song: "Durga" by Janet Stone and DJ Drez

Practices That Work with Your Theme

Offer poses that allow students to face fears: arm balances and inversions.

Distill Your Theme to a Short Sentence or Intention

Embrace your bravery.

Phrases or Sentences to Employ in These Parts of Your Class

OPENING	DURING MOVEMENTS
Fear is an emotion of self-caretaking. It crops up when there is risk! We can use fear to help us determine whether we should avoid something because we may be in real danger or whether there is reward to the risk. We'll play with poses today that allow us to find that reward.	As you practice this next shape, allow yourself to feel nervous. And then try it anyway.
DURING PAUSES	**CLOSING**
How does it feel to have pushed past your fear?	Notice the confidence that challenging your fears has imbued in you.

Takeaway Ideas

Because we associate large cats with courage in the face of fear, you could gift your students lion and tiger stickers as talismans of their bravery.

Anything Else

You might share with your students that Durga is just one manifestation of Shakti; she's part of a divine whole. Just like Durga, your students' fear, courage, and bravery are only small parts of their essential wholeness.

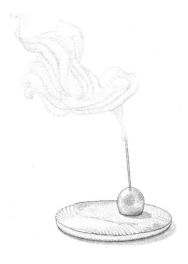

10

SHIVA AND SHAKTI: THEMES FROM THE MASCULINE AND FEMININE DIVINE

One of our favorite experiences in yoga has been yoga dance. We've most often gotten to enjoy this practice at Kripalu Center for Yoga and Health, but we're lucky enough to have a skilled practitioner who offers it at Sage's studio from time to time. If you've never experienced this joy of free-flowing, guided movement, we encourage you to try it: It's powerful yoga, but also very different from a typical yoga class where poses are cued and called out. Instead, in the practice of yoga dance, the teacher may offer movements that can be mirrored or mimicked, followed by options to dance to the music in your own way. Sometimes in yoga dance, you partner with another dancer—a beautiful opportunity of connection with others. We've often been moved to tears during this practice, as we unlock parts of ourselves that have been aching for the expression of dance!

One of the most powerful explorations in yoga dance is when the teacher asks you to imagine yourself in a certain role, and then you dance from that role. You may imagine you are at your most vulnerable and open, and dance from that place. You may imagine you are at your most powerful, and dance from that place. Getting to imagine yourself in these roles and then *moving* from that place is where the magic happens. What does it mean not just to imagine yourself as powerful but to move your body from a place of power, as a tool for power, with the fullness and confidence of your own greatness? We love these next themes of Shiva and Shakti, and you'll notice we approach them in this similar way: of offering students an opportunity to embody these masculine and feminine parts of themselves that may be lying dormant, waiting for this chance at expression in a safe space.

You might reassure your students that they don't need to identify as male, female, or nonbinary to appreciate these archetypes. We both identify as female, and we love to explore and feel the masculine energies of Shiva move through our bodies in movement.

FOR MORE

More Themes to Explore

Theming on archetypes of the feminine and masculine is nearly infinite. There is so much to explore here! More theming on Shiva and Shakti could take you on a journey of discussing consciousness and energy, the more ethereal forms of these deity figures.

Reading

The dichotomy of Shiva and Shakti is at the heart of Tantra Yoga. Georg Feuerstein's *Tantra: The Path of Ecstasy* (Boston: Shambhala, 1998) and Daniel Odier's translation of the *Yoga Spandakarika: The Sacred Texts at the Origins of Tantra* (Rochester, VT: Inner Traditions, 2005) are great places to start to learn more.

···· SHIVA: BECOMING THE PROTECTOR ····

Expound on Your Theme and Connect It to a Personal and a Universal Experience

Shiva embodies many roles, and one of them is protector. In one myth, Shiva helps the sacred river Ganges remain calm enough that humans could continue to use the water there without fear of drowning. Shiva's protective weapon is his *trishul,* or trident, which he is often depicted with.

Consider when you embody the role of protector. Are you protective of your children? Your partner? Do you walk in the world with an identity that means you must be protective of yourself? Does offering protection for yourself and loved ones come easily? Where are you most in need of protection? From whom or what? In a themed class on Shiva as protector, students get a chance to channel their inner Shiva to find the protection and strength as they navigate the world.

Chants, Quotes, Mantras, Poems, or Songs That Connect

Song: "Shiva (Supreme Soul)" by MC Yogi

Song: "Thrill of It All" by Satsang

Practices That Work with Your Theme

Standing Star Pose is a powerful pose of protection.

In any standing poses where the arms are raised overhead, cue students to practice *Kali mudra,* fingers clasped, index fingers outstretched, left thumb over right. This mudra suggests fearlessness!

Offer a guided meditation where students visualize a force field around them.

Distill Your Theme to a Short Sentence or Intention

Today, your protector awakens.

Phrases or Sentences to Employ in These Parts of Your Class

OPENING	DURING MOVEMENTS
As we move today, move your body as if you are ready to protect the most sacred beings that you love: your family, your friends, your community, yourself.	Can you move into this pose, fuller, more confident, more ready to stave off attacks and hold your ground?
DURING PAUSES	**CLOSING**
In this place of rest, you can let your guard down, knowing your barriers are reinforced, your protections are in place, and you are safe.	Notice how embodying your full protective power has awakened its greatness inside of you. Walk into the world with this new confidence, this new sense of safety.

Takeaway Ideas

You could offer your students trishul talismans—these could be small trident-shaped beads, or even lightly sketched trishul images they could take with them. Or, if you offer a guided meditation of visualizing a force field, record it and send it to your students after class.

Anything Else

If students seem reluctant to try on a new protective identity during the practice, know that that's OK. Even if they don't seem to embody it, they are hearing that they can be powerful and strong: That's an excellent starting place!

···· SHIVA: THE PEACEFUL WARRIOR ····

Expound on Your Theme and Connect It to a Personal and a Universal Experience

Real power doesn't bluster. A powerful warrior doesn't hesitate. A strong presence is steady and controlled. Without preening or bragging, deeply brave and courageous people exude confidence. Consider: Is there anything sexier than when someone embodies both strength *and* calm?

Power is action, not empty talk *about* action. To move as a peaceful warrior, invite students not to hesitate, but also not to rush. Embodying the peaceful warrior means to be certain you have the weapons of warfare at your disposal without needing to unnecessarily employ them as evidence.

As you imagine yourself as a peaceful warrior, you may be a warrior for love or social justice. You may imagine yourself a peaceful warrior in a toxic workplace or as you navigate challenging familial relationships. In these places, can you operate strategically from a place of strength and calm?

Chants, Quotes, Mantras, Poems, or Songs That Connect

Song: "Live Like a Warrior" by Matisyahu

Song: "Inner Peace" by Beautiful Chorus

Aphorism: *Si vis pacem, para bellum:* If you desire peace, prepare for war.

Practices That Work with Your Theme

Have students move in and out of Humble Warrior Pose, alternating between bowing and standing tall.

Cue students to arrive in Warrior II Pose and close their eyes, finding the peace in their strong bodies.

Distill Your Theme to a Short Sentence or Intention

Know that you would win every battle.

Phrases or Sentences to Employ in These Parts of Your Class

OPENING	**DURING MOVEMENTS**
A peaceful warrior has focus, presence, and calm. Invite those feelings into your body before we begin to move. Your calm belies your fierce and certain power.	What does it mean to move into this challenging pose in a peaceful way? Can you find more control here? Can you slow down and move powerfully?
DURING PAUSES	**CLOSING**
Here, your physical calm matches your internal calm. Even here, your power doesn't wane or cease. You are resting, confident in your ability to rise.	Walk off your mat today more certain as you make your way in the world. You have nothing to prove about your own strength; own it.

Takeaway Ideas

Give students a note card that says, *"Si vis pacem, para bellum."*

Anything Else

We desire confident and certain leadership, not only from our internal selves but also from the leaders we elect to lead our cities, states, and countries. You might offer this theme during times of civic, state, or federal elections.

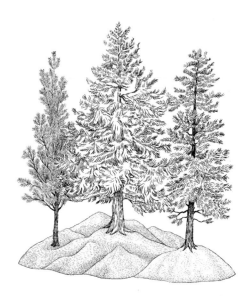

SHIVA: THE ARROW OF INTENTION

Expound on Your Theme and Connect It to a Personal and a Universal Experience

Sankalpa is your personal resolve or intention. We often use the word *intention* at the start of our yoga practice to suggest a philosophical or spiritual concept to focus on for the duration of the practice. But what about your prevailing intention off the mat? When you walk into the world, what heartfelt desire is guiding you as you manifest growth? Yogini and author Kathryn Budig has a book titled *Aim True,*[*] and we love that phrase, aim true, as the essence of this theme.

Shiva, the embodiment of consciousness, moves with clear intention. Our practice will offer a chance to emulate that single-pointedness.

Chants, Quotes, Mantras, Poems, or Songs That Connect

Song: "Satyam Shivam Sundaram" by Thievery Corporation

Chant: *Om namo bhagwate rudraay:* I bow to the almighty (the Shiva Rudra Mantra)

Practices That Work with Your Theme

Exploring versions of Warrior III—different arm variations, or different ways of coming into or out of the pose—would pair well with this theme.

Distill Your Theme to a Short Sentence or Intention

Rise, undeniable one. Aim true.

---

[*] Kathryn Budig, *Aim True: Love Your Body, Eat Without Fear, Nourish Your Spirit, Discover True Balance* (New York: William Morrow, 2016).

Phrases or Sentences to Employ in These Parts of Your Class

OPENING	DURING MOVEMENTS
Can you fill every shape today with the clarity of your intention?	To move with resolve means that you are not holding back; you are confident that you are exactly where you need to be. Can you feel that in your body here?
DURING PAUSES	**CLOSING**
Come back to your breath and come back to your truth. Here, you can cease the vigilance of aiming, knowing your intention is intact.	From this practice, bring with you the certainty of your purpose.

Takeaway Ideas

The imagery of an arrow is powerful. Include that in any small takeaway gift.

Anything Else

You might talk in more depth about the concept of sankalpa, or even share what guides your sure and unwavering arrow of intention.

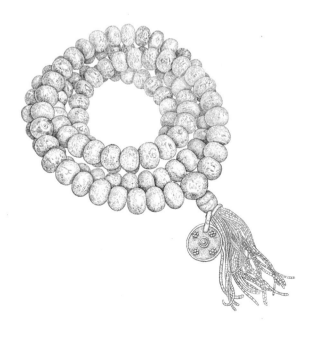

SHAKTI: EMBRACING THE CYCLES

Expound on Your Theme and Connect It to a Personal and a Universal Experience

Shakti reminds us to embrace, not resist, the cycles of life. We already discussed the cycle of creation-preservation-destruction, but cycles are everywhere. Shakti reminds us to lean into aging as another phase and place in life. Embracing the cycles allows us to see the value in the moodiness and heart-opening of premenstrual days, knowing the ease of release and renewal is coming. Shakti gives us permission to ride out the destructive moments, to see them not as an end but as part of an endless cycle of beginning again.

Shakti takes many forms, or avatars, in Hindu stories. Sometimes she is a fierce warrior, sometimes a patient wife, sometimes a mother, a daughter, and sometimes she sacrifices herself for others. Sometimes she demands sacrifices from others. She can embody cleanliness and purity, focused on the salvation of others. Or she can be a great destroyer, ridding the world of negative energy. Consider the roles you play and the cycles connected to those roles.

Chants, Quotes, Mantras, Poems, or Songs That Connect

Poem: "Go to the Limits of Your Longing" by Rainier Maria Rilke, especially the line, "Just keep going. No feeling is final."

Song: "Hurricane Waters" by Citizen Cope

Chant: The river is flowing, down to the sea.

Practices That Work with Your Theme

You might share how the three parts of a connecting vinyasa (Downward Dog, Plank to Chaturanga, Upward-Facing Dog or Cobra) can represent this cycle in action.

Distill Your Theme to a Short Sentence or Intention

Embrace the waves.

Phrases or Sentences to Employ in These Parts of Your Class

OPENING	DURING MOVEMENTS
Today as we practice, you get to move with absolute embrace of everything that arises, seeing it as necessary, as part of the greater whole. We'll practice embracing moments of ease and striving, and even little moments of success or failure, creation, and destruction in our movement practice.	Feel the cycle here: in your breath, in your movements, in your mental chatter that's narrating and commenting on your experience. It's all in flux, moment to moment, movement to movement. Ride the wave.
DURING PAUSES	**CLOSING**
This rest period is part of the cycle too. Without taking this downtime, we wouldn't have the energy to move skillfully through what's next. Lean in to this rest.	Think ahead at least one upcoming time cycle: this could be a day, week, month, or year. What will be different then? What will be the same? How does your practice keep you present, whatever comes?

Takeaway Ideas

Offer your students a little card with a line drawing of a wave.

Anything Else

The more we normalize the cyclical nature of emotions, personal growth, and life, the better! With your students, generalize the relevant aspects of the cycles you move through.

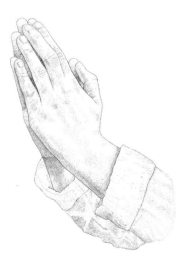

SHAKTI: DIVINE MOTHER

Expound on Your Theme and Connect It to a Personal and a Universal Experience

The divine *mata* is the personification of nurturing. In this incarnation of the goddess, caretaking is the guiding force. As you embody this nurturance, you get to see yourself as both nurtured and nurturing. How does it feel to be maternal? And how does it feel to receive this mothering at your own hands?

Chants, Quotes, Mantras, Poems, or Songs That Connect

Song: "Fruits of My Labor" by Lucinda Williams

Song: "Saraswati Mata" by Daphne Tse

Quote: "The common expression is 'I love you.' But instead of 'I love you,' it would be better to say, 'I am love—I am the embodiment of pure love.' Remove the *I* and *you,* and you will find that there is only love." —Sri Mata Amritanandamayi (Amma)

Practices That Work with Your Theme

Self-massage.

Include some restorative yoga poses (with props) before you move into Savasana.

Distill Your Theme to a Short Sentence or Intention

Nurture yourself from a place of abiding self-love.

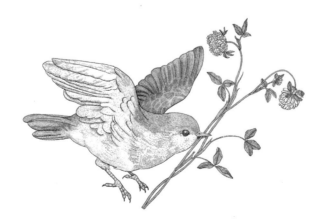

Phrases or Sentences to Employ in These Parts of Your Class

OPENING	DURING MOVEMENTS
As we prepare to move with this theme of divine motherhood, take a moment to consider your ideal maternal representation. This could be your own mother or grandmother—but if that proves problematic, think about someone you've witnessed parenting in a way that speaks best to you, in real life or on TV or in a movie or a book. Can you find a word or two to describe the essence of this nurturing? Then can you return to this word throughout the practice?	Remember the words you used to describe your ideal mother. Do they inform your movement here? What would this ideal mother say to encourage you in this moment?
DURING PAUSES	**CLOSING**
Here is another opportunity to nurture yourself, to mother your inner child. Make yourself comfortable here. Tuck yourself in.	Trust that you are held. You are held by the earth, by the divine. You are nurtured. You are loved.

Takeaway Ideas

The humanitarian activist and guru Amma is known as the "hugging saint." Hugging is life-affirming, nourishing spiritual practice. If you know your students well, offer them a hug after class.

Anything Else

Because students in a general class might have different relationships with their mothers—some warm, some challenging—it can be wise to talk about this theme in relation to maternal *energy*, not the manifestation of that in actual mothers.

If you're interested in the relationship between yoga and motherhood, read *Whole Mama Yoga: Meditation, Mantra, and Movement in Pregnancy and Beyond,* co-authored by Alexandra and our colleague Lauren Sacks (Boca Raton, FL: Health Communications, 2023). The book offers practical thought on prenatal and postpartum asana and explores the connection between the philosophy of yoga and the practice of being a mother.

···· SHAKTI: EMBODYING THE GODDESS ····

Expound on Your Theme and Connect It to a Personal and a Universal Experience

Channel your inner princess diva, your flamboyant drag queen, your high priestess of full and sassy radiance. Embody the goddess that has always been you.

In a practice on embodying the goddess, invite students to strut, to preen, to sway their hips, and seductively dance their yoga—all for themselves. The supreme goddess or Mahadevi embodies all: joy and exuberance, fierceness and play, sexy youth, and inspired wisdom. How does your inner goddess express herself? You may notice as you begin that at first, this feels silly or performative. You may feel like you are "playing at" being this audacious version of yourself. But look for the little moments when it starts to feel authentic, where you begin to recognize that this goddess resides inside you too.

Chants, Quotes, Mantras, Poems, or Songs That Connect

Song: "The Seductress" by Wynton Marsalis

Song: "Good as Hell" by Lizzo

Song: "Queen of Hearts (Radhe Radhe)" by Jai Uttal

Practices That Work with Your Theme

Bring your students into a familiar pose, and then ask them to embody it as a goddess. Model this yourself, perhaps cocking a hip or spreading your fingers. What does being radiant feel like? Show that to your students so they can find it in themselves.

Distill Your Theme to a Short Sentence or Intention

Seduce yourself.

Phrases or Sentences to Employ in These Parts of Your Class

OPENING	DURING MOVEMENTS
You get to be a goddess in your practice today. Does that idea scare you or enliven you? Whether it makes you nervous or intrigues you, commit to the bit. Find your inner goddess and let her out!	Can you be sassier here? Can you be bolder and more daring? Can you radiate as you arrive in this pose?
DURING PAUSES	**CLOSING**
When the goddess comes to rest, everyone knows it. Even here, take up space, and honor yourself in the stillness.	Strut off your mat and out of this room exuding divine goddess energy. Smile. Get your way. Own your power.

Takeaway Ideas

Bring a selection of bright nail polish to class, and invite your students to paint a finger or a toe (maybe just a pinky toe) a vibrant shade of fuchsia or magenta to remind them of their time as a yoga goddess.

Anything Else

People often associated Tantra yoga with sex. At the heart of this misnomer is that the *tantrikas* understood their existence on earth to be a playground for liberation. That meant they saw all human activity and inclination—including sexuality—as part of that.

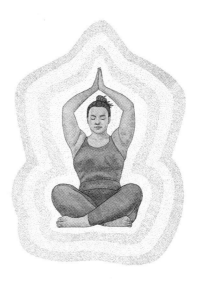

11

REBEL, YOGI!

Yoga is a radical practice. Its explicit goal is liberation. In recognition of the brave souls—yogis at heart—who seek to implement freedom from suffering, we offer these themes that speak to social justice and, hopefully, impel students to action.

As we mentioned in part 1, there's only so much you can do in the context of a regular yoga class. That doesn't mean you shouldn't do what you can: Don't turn away from injustice, and don't indulge in spiritual bypassing by leaning on "good vibes only." The first step to solving any problem is in acknowledging the problem. And that's exactly what happens in a good yoga class: You have a chance to see things as they are, to recognize the nature of a situation, and to experience yourself as the seer.

FOR MORE

More Themes to Explore

Protecting the vulnerable; vulnerable people need social attention.

Look for the helpers (a reference to the famous Mr. Rogers quote).

Vishuddha chakra and speaking truth

Sangha and the power of yoga community

Reading

Stephen Mitchell, *Bhagavad Gita: A New Translation* (New York: Harmony, 2000).

Michelle Cassandra Johnson, *Skill in Action: Radicalizing Your Yoga Practice to Create a Just World* (Boulder, CO: Shambhala, 2020).

Swami Vivekananda, *Karma Yoga,* https://archive.org/details/Karma YogaswamiVivekanandaBook.

Faith Hunter, *Spiritually Fly: Wisdom, Meditations, and Yoga to Elevate Your Soul* (Boulder, CO: Sounds True, 2021).

Jessamyn Stanley, *Every Body Yoga: Let Go of Fear, Get On the Mat, and Love Your Body* (New York: Workman, 2017).

Jacoby Ballard, *A Queer Dharma: Yoga and Meditations for Liberation* (Berkeley, CA: North Atlantic Books, 2021).

Heather Plett, *The Art of Holding Space: A Practice of Love, Liberation, and Leadership* (Vancouver, Canada: Page Two, 2020).

BLACK LIVES MATTER

Expound on Your Theme and Connect It to a Personal and a Universal Experience

How do we translate this well-known slogan to action on and off the mat? Yoga teaches sustained attention as limb six of the eight-limbed path. We call it *dharana*, single-pointed concentration. This is a critical skill for holding space to care for groups that need our care. The knee-jerk reaction "All lives matter" is but a selfish response to the recognition that Black family, friends, and neighbors need our care and attention to correct the systemic injustices that the United States—and Western culture writ large—was built on. Dharana teaches us to keep our attention where it needs to stay and not to flinch or turn away or try to center ourselves in the narrative.

Chants, Quotes, Mantras, Poems, or Songs That Connect

Poem: "Still I Rise" by Maya Angelou

Song: "Freedom" by Beyoncé

Quote: "If you are silent about your pain, they'll kill you and say you enjoyed it." —Zora Neale Hurston

Quote: "He who is rooted in oneness realizes that I am in every being; wherever he goes, he remains in me. When he sees all beings as equal in suffering or in joy because they are like himself, that man has grown perfect in yoga." —Bhagavad Gita 6.32, translated by Stephen Mitchell

Practices That Work with Your Theme

Practicing a *drishti* gaze, with single-pointed focus during standing poses.

Practice Surya Bhedana, Sun-Piercing Breath.

Distill Your Theme to a Short Sentence or Intention

Black lives matter. Keep your attention where it needs to stay.

Phrases or Sentences to Employ in These Parts of Your Class

OPENING	DURING MOVEMENTS
Our theme is a reminder that when any part of us suffers, we all suffer; that is the bargain of our shared humanity. Let's move our bodies with that knowledge fueling our practice.	You inherently know that your life matters here. You're moving in and out of poses with fluidity of movement with your breath as the drumbeat backdrop. You are safe here. Notice how that feels: to know you are safe.
DURING PAUSES	**CLOSING**
In this moment of stillness, offer a silent wish for peace and equality. Send that intention into the world.	How will you carry this intention off your mat and allow it to shape your actions in the world? What is a tangible way you can show that Black lives matter?

Takeaway Ideas

Black Lives Matter stickers or pins.

Anything Else

Because we continue to live in a world that does not keep Black bodies safe and sacred, this powerful phrase has transcended slogan. We hope one day this feels like a dated watchword, but today is not yet that day.

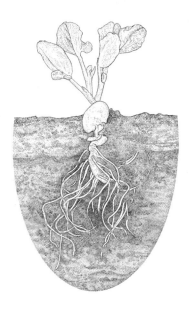

LOVE IS LOVE

Expound on Your Theme and Connect It to a Personal and a Universal Experience

The world needs more love in every format. Why do some people get hung up on the format part of this?

One lovely tool we learned from our friends who taught in the Anusara Yoga lineage is to always look for the good in others. This is called *sri* or *shri,* the exalted, higher self. The idea is similar to what we explored in "Lead with Your Heart" in chapter 7: It's to approach each interaction already looking for the good, for the noble, for the honorable in everyone you meet. When we operate from this heart-centered, good-oriented place, we lead with love. And by spreading more love, even in tiny bites, we venerate love in every form. We create more space for an abundance of love, and hopefully set the scene for all our students, who love in a broad variety of ways, to feel included and safe in yoga.

Chants, Quotes, Mantras, Poems, or Songs That Connect

Quote: "Have you ever loved the body of a woman? / Have you ever loved the body of a man? / Do you not see that these are exactly the same to all in all nations and times all over the earth?" —Walt Whitman, "I Sing the Body Electric"

Song: "True Colors" by Joshua Radin

Practices That Work with Your Theme

If it's appropriate for your population, partner yoga. Or even an exercise where you make eye contact, if only for a moment, with others in the room.

Distill Your Theme to a Short Sentence or Intention

Let love lead.

Phrases or Sentences to Employ in These Parts of Your Class

OPENING	DURING MOVEMENTS
When you love fully and openly, without reserve, you make space for others to do the same. Let your practice be a light of love, so that others may shine too.	Pause during your practice to look around for one moment. (We like to call this "Watchasana.") Freely offer love to all these beings around you, shining their lights. See the good in them.
DURING PAUSES	**CLOSING**
Feel your heart swell with love in this stillness.	This practice may have served as a love note to yourself. As you move off your mat, let your actions serve as a love note to people everywhere, and let your message be that all love is valid. All love is valid.

Takeaway Ideas

Any version of a rainbow, to signify your open-hearted support of the human rights of LGBTQIA+ people everywhere.

Anything Else

Pride month is a seasonally appropriate time to offer this theme, but be sure your students know it's your year-round practice.

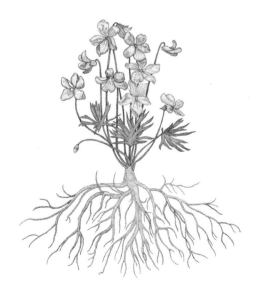

YOU ARE NOT A PRODUCT

Expound on Your Theme and Connect It to a Personal and a Universal Experience

Social media and visual culture—Instagram worst among them—seek to commodify yoga at every turn. It's depicted as a practice for thin white women in pricey clothes on expensive mats in exotic locales at sunset. When the message is that spending money will fast-track your practice, how can you decommodify your yoga?

A good first step is to remove the trappings of consumerism from your practice. Try practicing yoga in your pajamas—or, heck, in your underwear or your birthday suit (at home, of course!). Try forgoing your mat and instead do some of your practice on the carpet, and some on the floor. The less you rely on the outward signifiers of "yoga!" to define your practice, the more authentic your practice becomes.

Differentiate between the practice of yoga—one of ancient wisdom aimed at your liberation—and the industry that tries to *sell* yoga and wellness to you.

Chants, Quotes, Mantras, Poems, or Songs That Connect

Song: "Traffic in the Sky" by Jack Johnson

Song: "Everybody Wants to Rule the World" by Tears for Fears

Song: "Royals" by Lorde

Song: "Big Yellow Taxi" by Joni Mitchell

Practices That Work with Your Theme

Lead a sequence that requires no mat and no props. Standing sequences that don't put hands on the floor work well.

Distill Your Theme to a Short Sentence or Intention

Your soul is not for sale.

Phrases or Sentences to Employ in These Parts of Your Class

OPENING	DURING MOVEMENTS
As we move through this practice, let's aim to free our bodies and minds from the commercial culture that says we need to look a certain way, smooth our clothes in a certain way, or reach for the deepest expression of a pose.	Notice if you're feeling a need to perform here. Can you move for the joy of it, free from trying to match some version of this pose you saw in a clothing catalog or on Instagram? How would it feel to do this movement with no one watching?
DURING PAUSES	**CLOSING**
You are not doing this practice for anyone but you.	What does it mean to be a yogi? When you aren't signaling yoga to the world in spandex fitness clothes or with beaded bracelets, what does your authentic yoga off the mat look like?

Takeaway Ideas

Offer your students little stickers or note cards that say "yoga deinfluenced" or "yoga deinfluencer."

Anything Else

With your students, continue to differentiate the practice of yoga, which is extremely personal, from the product of yoga, which is sold in every mala, harmonium, crystal, and essential oil that the wellness industry thinks you'll buy.

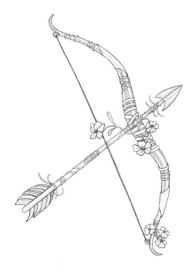

EQUALITY FOR ALL

Expound on Your Theme and Connect It to a Personal and a Universal Experience

The Sanskrit word that means equality or evenness is *sama*, a cognate for "same." You'll hear it in various iterations in a yoga class: in the description of Mountain Pose as Samasthiti, or "even standing"; the chant *Lokah samastha sukhino bhavantu*, where it appears as part of *samastha*, meaning "equally" or "all beings." Once we are listening for it, we hear it! And it's right there in the eighth limb of yoga: *samadhi*, equal seeing—which brings us bliss.

When we recognize ourselves in others, we can see and feel this sameness and equality. We get a little hit of it when we see someone delighting in the things that delight us, whether it's a flavor, a color, or a song. Sometimes it feels like a surprise when we see our sameness in others, but shared humanity is the rule, not the exception. We are all in this together.

Chants, Quotes, Mantras, Poems, or Songs That Connect

Song: "Free" by Florence + the Machine

Song: "Prayer of Peace" by Beautiful Chorus

Poem: "Goodbye to Tolerance" by Denise Levertov

Practices That Work with Your Theme

Balance poses. Point out to your students that balancing from one side to the other may feel very different, but we treat the experience the same.

Distill Your Theme to a Short Sentence or Intention

Your humanity is shared.

Phrases or Sentences to Employ in These Parts of Your Class

OPENING	DURING MOVEMENTS
Take a moment to look at your neighbor, your equal in this world. Say hello before we begin.	Notice that we are all moving and breathing in unison. Your personal experience on the mat is part of this greater whole.
DURING PAUSES	**CLOSING**
Can you hear your neighbor breathe? Can you feel the bodies of others in the room with you? As you rest, so do those around you.	Before you leave, say good-bye to someone in the room. Wish them a good day. Ask them where they're heading next. Before you leave, connect.

Takeaway Ideas

At the start of class, pass around a ball of yarn, and ask everyone to hold on to it. Note the symbolism of this tangible connection. As your students move, cut the yarn into lengths and give your students a length to take with them to remind them of this connection.

Anything Else

Even encouraging your students to know one another, like introducing them before class, is a way to increase community and help your students connect to their shared humanity. Consider more ways you can grow that connection. With your students' permission, you could unblind your email list so students could more easily connect with each other, for instance.

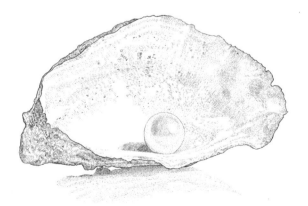

CHANGING THE THINGS YOU CANNOT ACCEPT

Expound on Your Theme and Connect It to a Personal and a Universal Experience

Reinhold Niebuhr's famous "Serenity Prayer," a mantra for twelve-step programs, says "God grant me the serenity to accept the things I cannot change, courage to change the things I can, and wisdom to know the difference." This maps on to the last three niyamas: *tapas, svadhyaya,* and *ishvara pranidhana.* Tapas, intense devotion, is about courage. Ishvara pranidhana means surrender to the divine, and thus serenity to accept what you cannot change. And svadhyaya, self-study, helps you build the wisdom to know the difference between the two. We often discuss this as a manual for your practice: Yoga asana gives us a chance to recognize what is changeable, and then discern whether it's worth changing. And at the same time, yoga gives us tools for accepting what we can't change.

But Angela Davis's famous quote turns this reading on its head: "I am no longer accepting the things I cannot change. I am changing the things I cannot accept." What a lovely upending! This flip of the concept reminds us that we have agency, and do not need to—should not—passively accept the unacceptable elements of our society and laws. Instead, we should rise up and use our courage for collective action in the service of building a better society.

And our practice gives us tools to make us agents of change: a sense of personal efficacy and strength; the ability to stay focused and present even in uncomfortable situations; a recognition of our place in the grand scheme of things.

Chants, Quotes, Mantras, Poems, or Songs That Connect

Mantra: I am strong. I matter.

Song: "I Can Change" by Lake Street Dive

Practices That Work with Your Theme

Challenging—but doable!—poses like Warrior III that build your students' confidence in their abilities.

Repetition of moves so that students can feel like they are moving toward mastery.

Distill Your Theme to a Short Sentence or Intention

Don't take it lying down.

Phrases or Sentences to Employ in These Parts of Your Class

OPENING	DURING MOVEMENTS
As we move into our practice today, consider some situation where you saw injustice being done and felt impelled to act. What tools helped you then? How can your practice today help sharpen those skills for you?	If you didn't feel like you nailed that shape on the first pass, that's OK. Let's do it again! Let this next foray into the shape be a chance for you to change the experience into something that affirms your strength and your ability.
DURING PAUSES	**CLOSING**
Use your breath to recenter here. Let this downtime be a gathering of your energies, so you can move into the next sequence ready to create positive change.	As you prepare to move off the mat and back into the world that can feel quite broken, can you focus on one issue where your skills could create positive change? Name to yourself the first next step to take. Recognize the ways your practice has helped to make you an agent of change.

Takeaway Ideas

If there's a volunteer experience your students could undertake individually or together, from roadside cleanup to mentoring at-risk youth, give them the details about how to help.

Anything Else

Do the work, and share with your students the ways you are working to change things you can no longer accept.

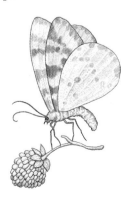

INTERDEPENDENCE

Expound on Your Theme and Connect It to a Personal and a Universal Experience

No man is an island, as John Donne so beautifully wrote in his poem of that name. Instead, "Every man is a piece of the continent / A part of the main." No matter how lonely you might feel on a tough day, your existence depends on—and feeds in return—everyone around you. The infrastructure of our society is the dependence we have on each other doing any task, from driving to dressing to eating.

Once we recognize this interdependence, we realize we are not alone. And we are called to compassion for all of humanity, since, as Donne wrote,

Any man's death diminishes me,
Because I am involved in mankind,
And therefore never send to know for whom the bell tolls;
It tolls for thee.

A benefit of the yoga practice is feeling this sense of connection, compassion, and sympathy. Yoga means union; when we practice, we unite body, mind, and spirit. And when we practice in community we unite with each other, even just by sharing air as we breathe.

Chants, Quotes, Mantras, Poems, or Songs That Connect

Song: "Lean on Me" by Bill Withers

Song: "Think" by Aretha Franklin

Song: "Wildflowers" by the Wailin' Jennys

Quote: "I am involved in mankind." —John Donne

Practices That Work with Your Theme

Group and partner poses: Tree Pose or Warrior III in a circle facing inward, hands on your neighbors' backs.

Using a partner to rise from sitting to standing: Face each other and hold each other's wrists so you can rise up easily, or sit back-to-back for a challenge.

Any chanting; breathing at a volume that reminds students they are in a group.

Distill Your Theme to a Short Sentence or Intention

I need you. You are not alone.

Phrases or Sentences to Employ in These Parts of Your Class

OPENING	DURING MOVEMENTS
At its best, the yoga practice shows us that all things are connected. When we hit the flow state yogis call samadhi, we feel a blissful connection. We can't force that state, but we can invite this sense of connection in today by recognizing the ways we depend on each other. See if you can bring your breath up to a volume that reminds your neighbors that we are here together—but not so loud that you can't hear them sending the same message to you.	As we play with this partner movement, feel the power you get from each other. How does leaning on each other lighten the load?
DURING PAUSES	**CLOSING**
As you settle into this rest shape, can you feel the presence of your classmates? Where in your body are you aware of our community? Is it your ears, your hands against the floor? Your heart?	Think ahead to a need you can fill, perhaps using a skill or resource you have available and can share with a neighbor. This can be as simple as listing some giveaways on the local buy-nothing group, or as big as donating your time or money to a local cause. Now plan the first next step toward sharing your gifts.

Takeaway Ideas

If your students are familiar with each other and your studio allows, take a group photo after class and share it!

Anything Else

If you have a regular class of students who all know each other, you could offer this theme in connection to some light partner yoga.

12

LESSONS LEARNED FROM OUR STUDENTS

We learn as much from our students as they do from us—and maybe more. It's especially illuminating to hear how the messages we deliver in class, intentionally or unintentionally, land with our students. Here are some of the sweetest themes or lessons that have been shared with us.

FOR MORE

More Themes to Explore

Ask your students for their go-to themes! What mantras or intentions do they commonly set? Not only will you get to know your students more, but you'll also find beautiful new avenues of inspiration from the people who come to your classes.

Reading

Instead of offering suggestions for reading here, we'll remind you that talking openly with others about what inspires you frees them to share what inspires them!

YOU DON'T KNOW YET WHEN THIS PRACTICE WILL COME IN HANDY

Expound on Your Theme and Connect It to a Personal and a Universal Experience

One of our studio regulars turned up after an absence, when she'd been caring for her mother after her mother had a stroke. "All my movement practices have been so helpful," she said. She was using her awareness of core strength, martial arts, and yoga asana to lead her mother's rehab, and of course her mindfulness was critical throughout.

This made us think about why we practice: It's so we can draw on the practice when the rubber hits the road off the mat—in caring for others, in coming back to center, in maintaining grace under pressure. While you may come to the mat to develop these skills in response to an ongoing problem you face, you'll inevitably encounter new problems. You may not know yet why you are practicing.

Chants, Quotes, Mantras, Poems, or Songs That Connect

Chant: *Om namah shivaya:* I bow to the inevitability of change.

Song: "Love Holding Love" by Wah!

Song: "Don't Give Up" by Peter Gabriel with Kate Bush

Practices That Work with Your Theme

Any bowing or forward folding.

Any challenging pose that requires you to develop skill to stay present even when things are hard.

Every transition from low to high and back again.

Distill Your Theme to a Short Sentence or Intention

This will help you in ways you don't see yet.

Phrases or Sentences to Employ in These Parts of Your Class

OPENING

Sometimes doing yoga practice can feel like learning calculus as a required class: "When am I *ever* going to use this?" As we develop new skill and expertise on the mat today, recognize that it will help in ways you can't even see yet.

Try thinking back to a time in your life when you used a lesson from yoga off the mat. It could be as simple as remembering to take a few deep breaths before heading into a meeting or a challenging conversation, or systematically relaxing your body before you fall asleep.

DURING MOVEMENTS

Can you feel how the second round is easier than the first? Practice confers skills for greater ease in any situation.

Consider how the work you are doing here and now might be preparing you for traversing an icy sidewalk, picking up a child, or staying cool through air turbulence.

DURING PAUSES

Your body and mind adapt to learning new things during the rest. Take this downtime so you can learn better.

It's important to rest when you can, since in life you never know when something disruptive will come along and demand your energy and attention. Take this time to bank a few calm breaths.

CLOSING

One thing we practice in every class is how to greet the end we all have coming. How can you let go gracefully in Savasana?

Anticipate a challenge you expect to encounter in the next days or weeks. This could be a long run, a long drive, a long conference at work. Think of a movement or a phrase from today's class that might be useful in keeping you focused and grounded as you meet this challenge.

Takeaway Ideas

A written practice (for example, just a few gentle stretches or a restorative pose) for relaxing at the end of a challenging day.

A mantra for caregivers.

Anything Else

If it suits the vibe of your class, you might invite a short discussion about when students have found themselves using yoga tools in their daily lives. If this happens at the start of class, you can then call back to these moments as you go through the practice. And if your class is conversational, you can ask, "How does this shape mimic something you do in daily life?"

···· WHEN THE STUDENT IS READY, THE ···· TEACHER WILL APPEAR

Expound on Your Theme and Connect It to a Personal and a Universal Experience

Both of us have experience leading yoga teacher trainings and continuing education workshops. In the context of these trainings, students often have a pivotal story to share about why they decided to take the training. Indeed, Alexandra found yoga during a particularly hard chapter in her life, when a long-term relationship had come to a spectacular and heart-wrenching end. But the vulnerability required to navigate a challenging life event meant that she was ready, open, and prepared for the rigor of self-study and practice that yoga teacher training demanded. We bet you have a similar story about how you found yourself embracing yoga or how you arrived in the role of the teacher: Something in your life gave way to allow you to find the path. Consider that your readiness—whatever caused it—is the impetus. And then your teacher appeared.

Students arriving in a yoga class have a reason to be there, and they are signaling their openheartedness, their readiness, by their very presence. Maybe they're waiting for you as their teacher. Or maybe they're listening for a deep voice inside them to emerge as a teacher. Regardless, they are ready to learn.

Chants, Quotes, Mantras, Poems, or Songs That Connect

Song: "Learning to Fly" by Tom Petty and the Heartbreakers

Song: "You Learn" by Alanis Morissette

Chant: *Om Om Om gurur brahma gurur visnur gurur devo mahesvarah, guruh saksat param brahma tasmai sri-gurave namah* (Guru mantra or invocation: salutations to the great guru)

Practices That Work with Your Theme

Have students practice *padma mudra* (lotus hands, a reminder that beauty blooms from mud) in seated meditation.

Offer poses that stimulate the crown chakra, like Rabbit Pose and Headstand.

Distill Your Theme to a Short Sentence or Intention

When you're ready, everything is the teacher.

Phrases or Sentences to Employ in These Parts of Your Class

OPENING	DURING MOVEMENTS
Practicing yoga is an act of arrival, surrender, and readiness all at the same time. You are here to learn about yourself, about your place in community, about others around you. Welcome.	What can you learn from this pose? This transition?
DURING PAUSES	**CLOSING**
Notice the readiness in you. Showing up to your practice signals your desire to learn, to grow.	Leave class today with the clarity that you are ready to grow and ready to turn inward on your journey.

Takeaway Ideas

A little note card that says "You're ready."

Anything Else

"When the student is ready, the teacher will appear" is a familiar quote, but its roots are murky. It has been attributed to the Buddha, and the internet abounds with suggestions that it's from the Tao Te Ching (it's not). Despite not having a certain attribution, it has staying power because it rings true.

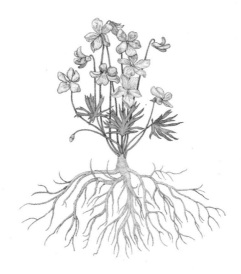

BE JOYFUL THOUGH YOU HAVE CONSIDERED ALL THE FACTS

Expound on Your Theme and Connect It to a Personal and a Universal Experience

"Be joyful though you have considered all the facts" is a line from Wendell Berry's poem "Manifesto: The Mad Farmer Liberation Front." The message of this theme is to live well and choose to spread joy *despite* knowing the dark truths and sadnesses that are part of existence. The model of our reality is entropy, and we know that in the end, the house takes all. In the face of this knowledge we can weep or be angry—or we can live on joyfully.

We were alerted to this lovely poem when one of our online students tagged us in a social media post where she used this quote as her theme. What a call to action it is! It is a reminder that despite what you know of the suffering of the world, you must live and love.

Chants, Quotes, Mantras, Poems, or Songs That Connect

Poem: "Manifesto: The Mad Farmer Liberation Front" by Wendell Berry

Song: "Northern Lad" by Tori Amos

Chant: *Om paranandaaya namah:* I am one with happiness.

Practices That Work with Your Theme

Have your students explore a challenging pose, like holding Plank, and invite them to laugh, smile, or express joy from that place.

Distill Your Theme to a Short Sentence or Intention

Be joyful.

Phrases or Sentences to Employ in These Parts of Your Class

OPENING	DURING MOVEMENTS
I don't know the facts of your day today. Maybe it has been one of ease or one of suffering. But despite your day, you are here now. Let that offer you a moment of happiness.	Even in moments of effort or challenge, there is joy to be found. Connect with that here.
DURING PAUSES	**CLOSING**
Is there more space for joy here amidst your breath?	As you move off the mat, how and when do you anticipate being able to find joy in the face of all the facts? What cue can you give yourself now to help remember this joy is available?

Takeaway Ideas

One sweet way to keep your students in a joy mind-set is to offer essential oil. You could include this as part of your Savasana assist, if you offer touch during your classes, or you could offer your students a spritz on their mats before or after class. (Make sure you know what oils should not be applied to the skin, and regardless, make sure any essential oil is diluted. Lavender oil is a safe bet!)

Anything Else

This theme is a light take on the philosophical shift from nihilism to absurdism. Those are concepts you could explore in further classes.

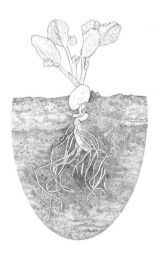

YOU ARE THE EXPERT ON YOU

Expound on Your Theme and Connect It to a Personal and a Universal Experience

Sage has a long-term student, Frank, whose athletic training was plagued with recurrent injuries. It all seemed to tie in to his right quadriceps, and much of what he tried to do to address the problem helped for a while, then reverted. In conversation with a friend who had just had ear surgery, he realized the issue might be tied to the bones in his inner ear, which had fused, changing the feedback he was getting from his vestibular system. Lo and behold: One simple surgery to his ear, and the issues began resolving. He had to work to adapt to this new sense of where his body is in space, but his injuries have abated and his performance has improved, even into his sixties. Frank saw his body as an *n* of one—that is, as a sample on which he could experiment to find out what might work best.

Unless a yoga teacher has carefully studied the latter books of the Yoga Sutras and developed some of the *siddhis,* the supernatural powers that it describes, they don't have x-ray vision to see inside a student and know what the optimal alignment is for that student. Only the student is the expert.

Chants, Quotes, Mantras, Poems, or Songs That Connect

Song: "Let Me Be" by Xavier Rudd

Song: "One for Me" by Khushi

Song: "Make Me Feel" by Janelle Monáe

Practices That Work with Your Theme

Offering frequent breaks and a host of different variations for each pose.

Give some broad cues: "Put most or all of your weight in one leg. Try lifting up some or all of the other foot. Find something fun to do with your hands." Or: "See if you can find three different ways to move to standing from here." Then let your students freestyle.

Distill Your Theme to a Short Sentence or Intention

You're the boss.

Phrases or Sentences to Employ in These Parts of Your Class

OPENING	DURING MOVEMENTS
Take the time to consider what brought you to practice today. And think also about your raw materials—how your body, breath, and mind are feeling right now. Marry your purpose with how you're feeling and set an intention that is unique to you.	Remember your intention. How can it guide you through this movement? Is changing something more in alignment with your intention?
DURING PAUSES	**CLOSING**
Come back again to your breath. Feel the uniqueness of your being. Decide what your one-of-a-kind body needs next.	Think ahead to a decision you might need to make in the near future. Is there something you learned about yourself from this practice, your study of one, that might help?

Takeaway Ideas

If your students have their phones handy, ask them to take a selfie on the way out of class. Encourage them to see the beautiful individuality in the picture. And tell them: "This is your real teacher."

Anything Else

As part of your approach to this theme, journal and investigate your relationship to yourself as your primary teacher.

MOVEMENT OPTIMISM

Expound on Your Theme and Connect It to a Personal and a Universal Experience

A healthy new trend in yoga instruction is turning away from don'ts and fear-based language—"Don't put your foot on your knee in Tree Pose!" for example—and instead offering a positive view of how capable, resilient, and changeable bodies are. It's called "movement optimism." We love this approach for several reasons.

First, as teacher trainees, we both had to learn a bunch of alignment rules, including a whole list of don'ts and contraindications. And then, as we taught real-world students, we had to unlearn virtually everything we had been taught. We came to realize that these rules get passed down from teacher to student because students believe their teachers have their best interests and safety at heart—and generally they do. So when students become teachers, they repeat the things they learned as students. Thus instructions that might have originally been created to achieve an aesthetic ideal of a shape, or that worked for fourteen-year-old boys or for dancer's bodies, get issued to a broad range of present-day students they were never designed for.

Movement optimism frees us from this cycle. It recognizes the ability inherent in every body. It decenters the teacher as the expert on how any pose should look or feel, and instead empowers the student to make the choices that work best for them, pose to pose, moment to moment. As such, this builds on our preceding theme, "You are the expert on you."

We can't think of a better message to give as teachers. And it's both totally personal—unique to each individual—and completely universal.

Chants, Quotes, Mantras, Poems, or Songs That Connect

Song: "Free to Be . . . You and Me" by the New Seekers

Song: "Free" by Kidswaste

Practices That Work with Your Theme

Fun transitions, like jumps forward or back, jump-throughs, and kicks to handstand.

Playful shifts to standing and back down to sitting, with suggestions like, "Try this with no hands this time!"

Distill Your Theme to a Short Sentence or Intention

Your body is strong, resilient, and able.

Yes, we can.

Why not?

Phrases or Sentences to Employ in These Parts of Your Class

OPENING	DURING MOVEMENTS
Can you think of a rule you've heard and maybe internalized? It could have to do with asana, or with anything you could imagine doing with your body. What if it weren't true?	Adopt the optimist's perspective. Imagine things going great. What if this transition goes well?
DURING PAUSES	**CLOSING**
Notice the approach you're taking here. Are you telling yourself the glass is half full, or half empty? What if you were just happy to have a glass of water at all?	Think how it would feel to adopt this optimism in other areas of your life—and not just the physical. What if you *could* do a pull-up? What if you *could* quit your job? What if you *could* find a partner who meets you where you are?

Takeaway Ideas

Give your students a note card at the start of class and invite them to write down yoga pose instructions and cues that they've heard that they don't understand or that don't work in their bodies. Take these cards back from them and address these cues and instructions over the course of future classes.

Anything Else

There are some wonderful yoga teachers talking about yoga and movement myths. One of our favorites is our friend and colleague Jenni Rawlings, who has a vibrant following on social media platforms.

CHOOSE WHAT TO BOMB

Expound on Your Theme and Connect It to a Personal and a Universal Experience

This theme came our way from a participant in one of Alexandra's Yoga for Motherhood retreat offerings. It's a profound theme on letting go in times of stress and overwhelm. Choosing what to bomb means mindfully, actively failing at some things. When we have multiple spinning plates in the air, it's inevitable one is going to drop and break. When you choose what to bomb, rather than watching things spin out of control, you opt early to fail. In practice, that may mean extending a deadline, getting takeout for dinner, or skipping leg day at the gym. This theme is a reminder that when we are overwhelmed or stressed, we can't do it all. And we don't have to.

Chants, Quotes, Mantras, Poems, or Songs That Connect

Song: "Let It Go" by James Bay

Song: "Bija" by Robert Rich and Lisa Moskow

Song: "Runnin'" by Frazey Ford

Practices That Work with Your Theme

Since this theme may be best employed at busy times, like the holiday season or back-to-school month, including a meditation practice during class time would work well.

If you play with balance or arm balance poses, invite students to explore to their edge and invite in "bombing" in the pose. In the case of arm balances, offer extra blankets for padded falls!

Distill Your Theme to a Short Sentence or Intention

Something has to give.

Phrases or Sentences to Employ in These Parts of Your Class

OPENING	DURING MOVEMENTS
You are allowed to give yourself what you need, even if it means you opt out of other things. Take that with you into our practice.	Let's try this shape, knowing we may bomb, inviting that in as part of the experience.
DURING PAUSES	**CLOSING**
Rest here. Maybe rest here for the remainder of the practice if opting out now allows you to care for yourself.	You are powerful. You are capable. You can employ wisdom as you choose what to mindfully fail at.

Takeaway Ideas

Give your students a little printout of the bomb emoji symbol as a reminder of this theme.

Anything Else

The parents of young children in your class may really relate to this one!

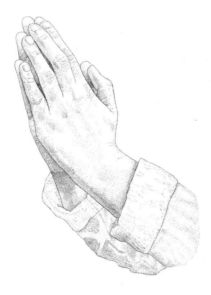

PART 3

JOURNAL PROMPTS AND TEMPLATES

13

NEW JOURNAL PROMPTS

The more you think through what matters to you, where you find inspiration, and what your purpose is, the better you can lead your students. And writing is a great way to practice since it encourages you to articulate your thoughts in ways that you can then carry right into the classroom. Or not! Your writing might be more exploratory. What matters is the practice of thinking through your role as a teacher and as a human being, then finding words to describe your thinking. Whether they ever make it off the page and into the studio is up to you.

In this chapter, we offer you some journal prompts. These are prompts that we have found especially helpful for harnessing our own voices at various points in our yoga-teaching journey. At https://teachingyogabeyondtheposes.com, you'll find these prompts collected for you in Word and Google Docs formats, so that if you like typing, you can respond right into your own file.

Where do you get hung up when planning class, and why do you think that is?

How do you add in the personal to share sophisticated ideas so that they come across as relatable, rather than lofty? Does that come easily for you?

Does the framework of yoga create the guiding principle of your life? If so, explain that. If not, explain what does guide your life. It may be a particular faith, or you may experience more a less-defined sense of spirituality. Regardless of that, it's helpful to understand your own core values, so write down what you know here. (This is a very helpful practice of svadhyaya, self-study!)

Who are your mentors or spiritual leaders? What do they believe? Are they living, available people you could have conversations with? Regardless, this exercise is useful. Make a list of the ideas you'd like to discuss with them or the questions you'd love to ask them.

What qualifies you to offer themes and philosophy on life? If this question makes you nervous, embrace that. That's an important starting point. Sit with that discomfort and marinate in it. Poke it. *Why* are you uncomfortable allowing your ideas to be elevated? *Why* do you doubt that you can lead others in ideas if you believe you can lead them in movement? How are those things different? Why is one scarier? And if this question doesn't make you nervous, embrace that! Has it ever made you nervous? If so, what changed?

We are unapologetically nonelitist about where our yoga class themes originate. All of life is a teacher. In reviews for *Teaching Yoga Beyond the Poses*, this was a point of contention for some readers. Even the most dedicated yogis surely watch a little TV or read lighter novels from time to time, don't they? Do we have to limit our inspirational materials to only ancient texts? For this exercise, stretch yourself to draw on something that you enjoy thoroughly but perhaps consider a guilty pleasure, like reality TV or video games, and find inspiration from that to share with your classes. Write a little about that here. Notice if you feel self-conscious about acknowledging your love of, say, pulp mysteries.

In our template, we ask you to consider what else connects to the theme and mention songs, quotes, poems, chants, or mantras. When you create themes, do you find that you tend to gravitate toward one of these more than others? Do you usually jot down a song? Do you feel more or less comfortable with poetry or mantras? Reflect a little on how you broaden your theme. Would you never chant? Do you feel comfortable reading or sharing poetry?

What unspoken beliefs do you have around *who* is allowed or qualified to offer spiritual, inspirational, or philosophical messages? Where do these beliefs come from?

Yoga and Hinduism blossomed in the same area of the world, and Hindu ideas and mythology weave through yoga. Are there any stories from Hinduism that you'd like to explore more?

What word, language, or phrase would you *never* use in a yoga class? Why? What would happen if you used that language or spoke these words to your students?

Do you ever feel like teaching movement, theming, controlling lighting and temperature, and maybe also doing something like curating a playlist or offering assists is too much happening at once? When that happens, what tends to get dropped?

Do smaller or larger classes make you a better teacher? Does class size change how you lead your class? How so?

In this book, you see how we have grouped our themes into chapters (for example, sutras, Shiva and Shakti, lessons from our students). Look at your own list of themes. What common threads do they have? If you were to apply categories and tags to them, what would they be?

What was your favorite theme of the fifty-four in this book? How would you add to it? What theme was confusing or didn't resonate, and why? How would you change that so it suits your brain and your students?

What message or theme do you come back to again and again? Why is this an important message for you?

If you take a yoga class and the teacher asks you to set your own intention, do you have a go-to or typical intention you set? Why or why not?

Can you think of a time you shared a message with your yoga class and you felt like your students connected to it? What did that feel like? And what made you think they connected to it so well?

Can you think of a time you shared a message with your yoga class and it felt like the message did not connect or land? What would you do differently?

14

TEMPLATES

THEME TITLE

Expound on Your Theme and Connect It to a Personal and a Universal Experience

Chants, Quotes, Mantras, Poems, or Songs That Connect

Practices That Work with Your Theme

Distill Your Theme to a Short Sentence or Intention

Phrases or Sentences to Employ in These Parts of Your Class

OPENING	DURING MOVEMENTS
DURING PAUSES	CLOSING

Takeaway Ideas

Anything Else

THEME TITLE

Expound on Your Theme and Connect It to a Personal and a Universal Experience

Chants, Quotes, Mantras, Poems, or Songs That Connect

Practices That Work with Your Theme

Distill Your Theme to a Short Sentence or Intention

Phrases or Sentences to Employ in These Parts of Your Class

OPENING	DURING MOVEMENTS
DURING PAUSES	CLOSING

Takeaway Ideas

Anything Else

THEME TITLE

Expound on Your Theme and Connect It to a Personal and a Universal Experience

Chants, Quotes, Mantras, Poems, or Songs That Connect

Practices That Work with Your Theme

Distill Your Theme to a Short Sentence or Intention

Phrases or Sentences to Employ in These Parts of Your Class

OPENING	DURING MOVEMENTS
DURING PAUSES	CLOSING

Takeaway Ideas

Anything Else

THEME TITLE

Expound on Your Theme and Connect It to a Personal and a Universal Experience

Chants, Quotes, Mantras, Poems, or Songs That Connect

Practices That Work with Your Theme

Distill Your Theme to a Short Sentence or Intention

Phrases or Sentences to Employ in These Parts of Your Class

OPENING	DURING MOVEMENTS
DURING PAUSES	**CLOSING**

Takeaway Ideas

Anything Else

THEME TITLE

Expound on Your Theme and Connect It to a Personal and a Universal Experience

Chants, Quotes, Mantras, Poems, or Songs That Connect

Practices That Work with Your Theme

Distill Your Theme to a Short Sentence or Intention

Phrases or Sentences to Employ in These Parts of Your Class

OPENING	DURING MOVEMENTS
DURING PAUSES	CLOSING

Takeaway Ideas

Anything Else

THEME TITLE

Expound on Your Theme and Connect It to a Personal and a Universal Experience

Chants, Quotes, Mantras, Poems, or Songs That Connect

Practices That Work with Your Theme

Distill Your Theme to a Short Sentence or Intention

Phrases or Sentences to Employ in These Parts of Your Class

OPENING	DURING MOVEMENTS
DURING PAUSES	CLOSING

Takeaway Ideas

Anything Else

THEME TITLE

Expound on Your Theme and Connect It to a Personal and a Universal Experience

Chants, Quotes, Mantras, Poems, or Songs That Connect

Practices That Work with Your Theme

Distill Your Theme to a Short Sentence or Intention

Phrases or Sentences to Employ in These Parts of Your Class

OPENING	DURING MOVEMENTS
DURING PAUSES	CLOSING

Takeaway Ideas

Anything Else

THEME TITLE

Expound on Your Theme and Connect It to a Personal and a Universal Experience

Chants, Quotes, Mantras, Poems, or Songs That Connect

Practices That Work with Your Theme

Distill Your Theme to a Short Sentence or Intention

Phrases or Sentences to Employ in These Parts of Your Class

OPENING	DURING MOVEMENTS
DURING PAUSES	CLOSING

Takeaway Ideas

Anything Else

THEME TITLE

Expound on Your Theme and Connect It to a Personal and a Universal Experience

Chants, Quotes, Mantras, Poems, or Songs That Connect

Practices That Work with Your Theme

Distill Your Theme to a Short Sentence or Intention

Phrases or Sentences to Employ in These Parts of Your Class

OPENING	DURING MOVEMENTS
DURING PAUSES	CLOSING

Takeaway Ideas

Anything Else

MAKE YOUR OWN TEMPLATE

At https://teachingyogabeyondtheposes.com, you can download templates to type into using your own preferred format—RTF, PDF, DOCX, and Google Docs. But we hope you'll use these as a starting point for adaptation to suit how *your* brain best works! That's the reason the template is free and editable.

Maybe you're a spreadsheet whiz, and color-coded cells keep you on track. Great! Perhaps you like writing your themes out by hand, with illustrations. Also great! We hope you'll riff on our basic template in whatever way will help you and your students best.

A note to those who are pen-and-paper types: every so often, snap photos of your carefully crafted themes, and sync them to your cloud service. That way, if you lose the paper version, you haven't lost the work.

If you like to track your themes and lesson plans on your computer or phone notes, consider adding #hashtags, categories, and tags for easier sorting and organization. At the very least, you might like to keep a running note file of what you taught to whom and how it felt, along with any feedback you received.

LET'S COLLABORATE

When you have themes that work especially well, we hope you won't hide them under a bushel, but instead share them with the yoga teaching community for everyone's mutual benefit. This can happen both locally—in your studio, your cohort of yoga teacher training graduates, and online. If you share your themes on social media, use the hashtag #teachingyogabeyondtheposes and tag us: we're easy to find. We'd also love to share your themes at https://teachingyoga beyondtheposes.com!

ABOUT THE AUTHORS

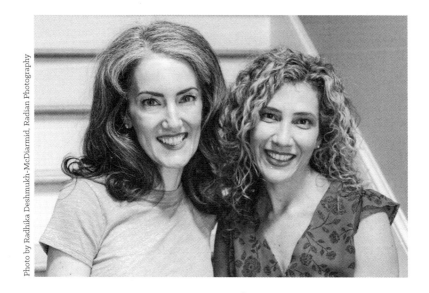

Photo by Radhika Deshmukh-McDiarmid, Radian Photography

Sage Rountree holds a PhD in English literature and the highest level of registration with the Yoga Alliance (E-RYT500, YACEP). She co-owns the Carolina Yoga Company and directs its two-hundred- and three-hundred- or five-hundred-hour teacher trainings. Sage has taught the same Monday-evening class there for more than twenty years. She also offers a robust virtual studio at https://sagerountree.com, including classes, teacher trainings, and retreats. Sage's work gives yoga teachers everything they need to feel confident, relaxed, and helpful in front of the classroom. Her most recent books are *The Art of Yoga Sequencing* (2024) and *The Professional Yoga Teacher's Handbook* (2020). She lives in North Carolina with her husband, Wes.

Alexandra DeSiato is an Experienced Registered Yoga Teacher at the highest level (E-RYT 500). She is also certified in Pilates and has an MA in English literature. Alexandra teaches and leads the two-hundred-hour yoga teacher training at Carolina Yoga Company. Find videos, blog posts, and more at https://alexandra desiato.com. Alexandra has partnered with Sage on two other books: *Lifelong Yoga* (2017), about healthy aging and yoga, and *Teaching Yoga Beyond the Poses* (2019), about yoga themes and inspiration. She is cocreator of a prenatal and postpartum yoga teaching collective Whole Mama Yoga (https://wholemamayoga.com), and she cowrote the yoga for motherhood guidebook *Whole Mama Yoga* (2023).

ABOUT THE ILLUSTRATOR

Lasha Mutual (https://lashamutual.com) is an artist whose deep commitment to Buddhist theory and practice has suffused her artistic expression, giving rise to a body of work that blends the action of painting with a meditative sense of contemplation and focus. Lasha's intention is to cultivate a generous, peaceful, and clear mind that becomes manifest in her artwork and that can be shared with others. She lives with her husband, son, and an abundance of pets in a little yellow brick cottage in Stratford, Ontario, Canada.

ABOUT NORTH ATLANTIC BOOKS

North Atlantic Books (NAB) is an independent, nonprofit publisher committed to a bold exploration of the relationships between mind, body, spirit, and nature. Founded in 1974, NAB aims to nurture a holistic view of the arts, sciences, humanities, and healing. To make a donation or to learn more about our books, authors, events, and newsletter, please visit www.northatlanticbooks.com.